Health Kinesiology

Jane Thurnell-Read

D1088235

Health Kinesiology

Jane Thurnell-Read
Life-Work Potential
Sea View House
Long Rock
Penzance
Cornwall TR20 8JF

Tel: 01736 719030

www.lifeworkpotential.com

Published by Life-Work Potential

Typesetting and production by:

ABLE PUBLISHING
13 Station Road, Knebworth
Hertfordshire SG3 6AP

Contents

Foreword

When I first met 'Isobel' she was about twenty. Her self-esteem was less than adequate - she smoked, ate junk food, and generally did not take good care of herself. Her older brother and his wife, my good friends, were unsuccessful at convincing her to change. The four of us were socializing once, when I discovered that Isobel was missing a little toe – amputated because of injury in an accident. She still had numbness and discomfort in the area, a classic 'phantom sensation'. With her consent I did a few energy corrections. Within about ten minutes all those symptoms had disappeared. For me, it was all very simple and routine. For Isobel, however, things developed rather unexpectedly. She returned home, quit her job, quit smoking, started eating 'real food', and moved to California. What had happened? That little bit of health kinesiology™ energy work with a 'nothing-can-be-done' condition had shown her that she could change. She could have control over her life. She had found hope.

In this book you will find numerous illustrations of how your own energy system is the key to the determination of precisely what is wrong or right for you and your body. In the world of the future I see treatment customized to each individual's specific needs. Gone will be the production line methods where everyone is given the same diet, drug, massage therapy, surgery, nutritional supplements, school program, exercise plan, or whatever. Furthermore, many of you will have learned how to do much of this for yourself. You will discover rather quickly that when you follow your body's true desires you will feel better, have more energy, be happier, be healthier, and function more effectively in every way.

Jane Thurnell-Read has given an overview of parts of my health kinesiology™ system and illustrated the procedures with dozens of real life examples. I hope that this book will inspire you to discover the same sort of life transformation, as have thousands of others. I have found no deeper satisfaction in my life than to see people overcome 'impossible situations' through my work. I thank Jane, and all of the people who have contributed, for helping you learn of the possibilities.

You can have the future now.

Jimmy Scott, PhD
Hastings, Ontario, Canada

Introduction

I became interested in kinesiology (from which health kinesiology developed) in 1981 when my eldest son, Jonathan, was just over a year old. He had chronic diarrhoea, eczema and was hyperactive, in spite of having a whole food diet. I knew what he was going through, as I had suffered with eczema since I was eight years old. As a teenager, when it was particularly bad, I would often wake with blood on the sheets, because I had scratched myself so badly in my sleep. Sometimes my eczema was so unbearable I would cry with the pain and the irritation. Conventional medicine had failed to provide a solution, and I had to some extent 'learnt to live with it'. I was determined that Jonathan should not suffer in his life, as I had. I knew I had to find some way to help Jonathan. I started reading various books on alternative medicine and allergies. Eventually I became convinced he was allergic to something, but none of the books offered a practical way of confirming that for a small baby.

In 1983 I went to the Festival of Mind and Body in London and came across a stand called Touch For Health. (This is a simplified version of applied kinesiology, mainly designed to allow lay people to deal with minor health problems. It can also be used preventively.) At the back of the stand there was a poster referring to something called 'muscle testing', and describing what it could be used for. This included allergies. I became very excited by this and, after talking to the people on the stand, took my son to see a touch for health practitioner based in London. Using muscle testing he found that Jonathan was allergic to wheat. I removed wheat from his diet and very quickly his eczema disappeared and his diarrhoea eased. I was thrilled and booked some sessions for myself. I was delighted to find that my own eczema started to clear too. Shortly after this I started touch for health training. Eventually I began to see clients and, not surprisingly, specialized in food allergies.

My second son, Thomas, was born with severe bronchial asthma. In order to help him I had to learn a lot about inhalant allergies and chemical sensitivities. This information proved extremely useful helping my clients too. I worked on my two sons regularly, and their health improved dramatically. When my youngest son was five years old, my new GP refused to believe he had ever had asthma because he was so well. He only became convinced that this was true when I named the consultant who had made the formal diagnosis.

Between 1983 and 1987 I tested several thousands of clients for suspected allergy problems. I had a very successful and busy practice, but I was becoming bored and frustrated, feeling that allergy problems were in fact a *symptom* indicating a further underlying problem. There are various other forms of kinesiology – applied kinesiology, three-in-one kinesiology, etc. – and I started to look at some of them. I also started learning about herbalism, iridology and homeopathy, but none of them seemed to be quite what I was looking for. Then, in 1987, I attended the first UK training course in health kinesiology, taught by its founder, Jimmy Scott.

I was very impressed: it seemed to be a thoroughly holistic system with a strong theoretical framework. I went home determined to try it out. I used Jonathan as the guinea pig: he had severe reading difficulties and had been diagnosed as dyslexic. Although he was eight years old, he read as though he had never met any of the words before. He was not very willing to allow me to practice on him, so we compromised with him lying on the sitting room floor watching television, while I scrabbled around with my new manual. I did not explain that I was trying to help his dyslexia, only that I wanted to try out some new techniques I had learnt. The session lasted less than an hour, with Jonathan repeatedly asking: "Haven't you finished yet?" That evening he read in phrases for the first time in his life. The benefit of that session lasted, and in the months that followed, as I learnt more advanced health kinesiology techniques, I did further work on him. His reading ability made further dramatic strides forward. From that very first session with my son I was immensely impressed by the power of this new kinesiology. From then on all my clients got HK, and I have never looked back.

I soon found that by using health kinesiology I could not only detect allergies, but could often correct the problems instantly. I also found that I could help people with a much wider variety of symptoms and problems both physical and psychological. I could also be very effective in helping people who were not ill, but who wanted help in achieving their potential.

I have now been practising HK for many years, and it never ceases to fascinate me. I am still amazed at the power, depth and breadth of HK, and its capacity to help people with a whole range of physical, psychological and spiritual problems.

Of course, the clients who stand out are the ones who benefited in a spectacular manner: the man in his seventies going blind whose sight improved so much after three sessions that he was able to drive his car again; the man who had suffered from depression for thirty years, and told me after one session: "The depression has completely gone; you cannot imagine the difference it has made to my quality of life", or the girl with severe epilepsy who is now fit-free and drug-free.

The miracle stories are, of course, very exciting and rewarding, but not everyone responds so quickly or dramatically. I gain a tremendous amount of satisfaction in helping people in less dramatic ways: people who need repeated appointments or who are less seriously ill, but who find that HK helps them overcome their problems and feel happier and more at peace with themselves.

When I started to write this book, I asked other HK practitioners for case stories. I was inundated with replies, and many of these marvellous stories are included in this book. There are many more that could not be included, if I were to produce a book of a manageable size. This avalanche of stories is a testament to the power of this therapy. Those included were chosen to illustrate a particular point and are not necessarily the most impressive. However, some of them may seem unbelievable, but they are all factual.

This is not intended as a comprehensive manual of all HK procedures for the student or practitioner. It is intended for the general reader who wants to understand more about this wonderful therapy.

Writing this book is partly a response to my sense of frustration that health kinesiology is not better known. Many people who would benefit from health kinesiology are not receiving it, not because they have rejected it, but because they do not even know it exists. I hope this book will bring the healing power of health kinesiology to many more people.

Jane Thurnell-Read

A glossary is included (see page 151 onwards).

1: What Is Kinesiology?

Kinesiology is the healing system from which health kinesiology developed. The word kinesiology means 'the study of movement' and was originally used to describe a field of medicine concerned with the working of joints and muscles. There are still people known as kinesiologists who work in conventional medicine, but, since the 1960's, other systems of kinesiology (including health kinesiology) have evolved from it.

The original work in this field was done by an orthopaedic surgeon, R.W. Lovett, in the 1920's. He developed a system for testing and grading the strength of muscles. This work was further developed and systematized by Henry and Florence Kendall, who published a book in 1949 entitled *Muscle Testing And Function*. In the early 1960's George Goodheart, an American chiropractor, developed this work further, when he realised that muscle weakness could often be rectified, at least temporarily, by massaging the beginning and end of the weak muscle, a procedure that came to be called the origin/ insertion technique. Goodheart also recognized that particular symptoms were often related to particular muscle weaknesses. He then integrated his insights with the work done in the 1930's by Frank Chapman and Terence Bennett. Chapman had found that, if he massaged certain tender places on the body, the area would stop being tender and people's health often improved. He related these to the lymph system of the body. The lymph system is part of the immune system of the body: massaging these points leads to an increased flow of lymph. Bennett found specific points (mainly on the head) that, when held, would lead to an increase in blood flow in the body. George Goodheart recognized that massaging Chapman reflex points and holding Bennett reflex points could also affect the response of the muscles. He now had three different ways of strengthening muscles: massaging the beginning and end of weak muscles, massaging points to increase lymph flow and holding points to increase blood flow. Goodheart also found that, if he worked to strengthen muscles, other health problems would improve or even disappear.

Acupuncture Meridians

He discovered that muscle response might be affected in ways that can only be explained by the traditional acupuncture theory of how the body works. According to this model there is a system of pathways or 'meridians' running up and down the body through which flows a 'vital energy' or 'life force' which drives and informs all the cells and functions of the body. If this energy system is in balance, health can be maintained. If it is disturbed, then physical or other disturbances may be produced or sustained. These energy disturbances also have an effect on muscle response, and the term 'kinesiology' has come to mean muscle testing to identify these disturbances.

The acupuncture meridians form part of the underlying energy system of the body. These were identified by Chinese practitioners thousands of years ago. They form a subtle energy grid that supports and integrates the different aspects of each individual: physical, emotional, mental and spiritual. The meridian energy system distributes Chi energy or life force to the body and this energy carries with it (or possibly even is) information to allow all the parts to function harmoniously. Imbalances in this system can lead to acute or chronic ill health as the life force energy or 'Chi' is not fed correctly to the tissues and cells of the physical body. When the meridian energy system is out of balance then this life force energy is not flowing properly.

In classical oriental medicine there are fourteen major meridian lines. There are two meridian lines on the midline of the body: the governing vessel running up the back of the torso, and the central or conception vessel running up the front of the torso. The other twelve meridians all run bilaterally on the surface of the body. These meridians are named after specific organs (e.g. the liver meridian, the small intestine meridian), but are not necessarily on or near the named organ. For example, the lung meridian runs down the inner arm to the thumb. The acupuncture meridians can relate directly to the health of the internal organ associated with it. The meridians are paired together into elements. Each pair consists of a yang meridian and a yin meridian. Yang meridians reflect qualities such as expansiveness, dryness, masculinity, lightness, heat and hollowness. Yin meridians reflect qualities of femininity, receptivity, darkness, coolness and solidity. The yang meridian needs its paired yin meridian for its completion. In HK the focus within the energy system is always on rebalancing the paired meridians.

Meridian Energy System Balance

The concept of balance is central to all branches of kinesiology. Kinesiologists believe that ill health is caused by imbalances within the system not only at a physical level but also emotionally and spiritually. Ideally the meridian energy system is in dynamic balance, changing and rebalancing according to internal and external circumstances. However, for many people the meridian energy is more often out of balance than in balance, leading to health problems. Many things can lead to imbalances in the meridian energy, including psychological stress, pollution, inadequate nutrition, etc. Kinesiologists work to redress these imbalances, so promoting good health and well-being.

There are points lying on the meridians which, if correctly stimulated, can overcome a disturbance and rebalance the energy system. Acupuncturists put needles into these points, but kinesiologists hold or rub combinations of points instead.

Muscle Testing

Muscle testing is a painless procedure involving the practitioner applying gentle pressure to specific parts of the body (often arms and legs) to test the response of the underlying muscle. The particular part of the body involved is placed in a specific position, in order, as far as possible, to isolate the muscle that is being tested. The muscle will either easily be able to resist the pressure from the practitioner or will give way, at least slightly. The kinesiologist uses this response to gain information about what is happening and what is needed to restore

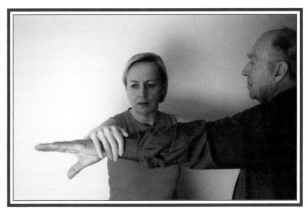

Muscle Testing

balance. Because of the inter-relationship between muscles, meridians and body systems, this information can apply not only to the muscle being tested but also give valuable information about other imbalances within the body and the necessary procedures to correct them.

Subtle Energy

Throughout this book you will see the terms **energy** and **subtle energy** used. This is not energy in the sense of calorie-energy. *The Concise Oxford Dictionary* defines **subtle** as: 'tenuous or rarefied … evasive, mysterious, hard to grasp or trace … making fine distinctions'. Subtle energy is a loose term used to describe any energy that is not specifically recognized and categorized by conventional scientific knowledge.

Some of these energies are seen as being part of man whereas others are seen as being outside of the individual person and are generated by completely separate sources.

In her book *Energy Medicine* Donna Eden describes this energy as: 'the common medium of the body, mind and soul. Its wavelengths, rates of vibration, and patterns of pulsation form their shared vocabulary.'

I can say with some certainty that subtle energy shares some of the characteristics of electromagnetic energy, but it is much more than this. This is a less than satisfactory explanation, but it seems that I am in good company. In *Scientific American* March 1999 George Musser writes: "Astronomers … can't find ninety per cent of the matter in the universe … Something swirls in the heavens and streams through our bodies without a whisper; it cannot be seen." He goes on to say that scientists have three different ways of weighing the universe and that "the discrepancies indicate that the universe is filled with some kind of extraordinary matter." It may be that this elusive matter is what alternative practitioners call 'subtle energy'.

Different Branches Of Kinesiology

All the different branches of kinesiology have originated from the work of George Goodheart. Because of its origins in physical therapy, applied kinesiology has tended to concentrate on structural problems and solutions. Other branches of kinesiology have been developed, including health kinesiology, educational kinesiology, classical kinesiology, creative kinesiology and 3 in 1 kinesiology. All use the basic muscle testing skills, but each kinesiology very much reflects the interests and personality of its developer. Some branches of kinesiology do not accept verbal muscle testing, which is a fundamental part of health kinesiology. Instead they rely on accessing information by testing a muscle whilst touching specific points on the body or using a finger mode. Finger modes are combinations of finger positions, which relate to specific body systems, correction procedures, and so on.

The muscle testing techniques of kinesiology have also been incorporated into other therapies. For example, homeopaths, Bowen practitioners, chiropractors and aromatherapists may use muscle testing to confirm their judgement about the correct course of action.

All kinesiologists are united by a fundamental belief and experience that each of us has an innate understanding of what is needed to become truly healthy. This information is at an other-than-conscious level and not easily accessible via the conscious mind, but it is accessible through the tool of muscle testing.

2: Introduction To Health Kinesiology

Health kinesiology was developed by Dr Jimmy Scott, amalgamating his own research and insights with that of other pioneers in the field of kinesiology.

In the early 1970s Dr Scott first saw a demonstration of muscle testing. At the time he was a psychologist, working as a research scientist at the University of California Medical School. He says: "I was both fascinated and highly sceptical." Over the next few years he saw further demonstrations of kinesiology. During this time he had become licensed as a psychologist and started to build up a practice in biofeedback and relaxation training. Eventually in 1975 he left the university and focused solely on his practice. Gradually he became more and more interested in the concept of 'health' and started to look to nutrition for answers. Again he

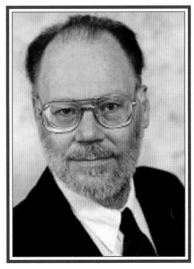

Jimmy Scott, the founder of HK

saw a demonstration of kinesiology by Chris Harrison, a chiropractor and diplomate of the International College of Applied Kinesiology. It was then that Jimmy began to realise the potential of kinesiology and started to attend kinesiology workshops. Very quickly he started to develop his own system: "my goals were to develop the most effective, robust, permanent methods for change that I could".

By 1981 the basic structure of the HK system was in place and further refinements and procedures were developed over the subsequent years. While HK is still evolving, the fundamentals of the system remain the same – they have stood the test of time. This impressive system of using a muscle response to access information is coupled with a range of powerful energy procedures that allow people to heal themselves. HK sees the individual as being a dynamic energy system encompassing physical, emotional, mental and spiritual attributes. In health kinesiology people are not viewed as physical bodies with inconvenient emotions tacked on.

Because the system accesses other-than-conscious information, the client does not need fully to understand why they have a problem when they consult a health kinesiologist, nor does the practitioner need an accurate medical diagnosis in order to proceed. The system does not depend on blind faith on the part of the client or placebo effect. Health kinesiology can also be used successfully for animals, although, sadly, in the UK it is illegal for anyone to work on an animal for money without the consent of a vet.

Bernhard Caspar is a health practitioner for animals in Germany and uses HK extensively in his work. Many of the Icelandic horses on the continent suffer from what is known as summer eczema. Bernhard has used HK with good results for these horses: in about sixty per cent of all the cases treated (nearly forty horses) he has been able to clear the problem immediately; for another twenty per cent he has been able to make a really measurable improvement. Bernhard is confident that, as he studies this problem more, his success rate will increase even further.

Health kinesiology practitioners work to help the client achieve balance and harmony. They work to help the physical body to become stronger and function better and to help clients feel happier, brighter and more fulfilled on every level of their lives. HK recognizes that, even where the symptoms manifest in the physical body, this may be because there are imbalances in the person's emotional life. For example, asthma, arthritis, vertigo or irritable bowel trouble may be reflecting disharmony and imbalance in the emotional, mental or spiritual areas. Sometimes work in one of these areas is all that is needed, because the physical problem is a reflection of imbalances elsewhere. The health kinesiology system also recognizes that the physical body **is** important, and that sometimes the best way to resolve physical symptoms is through nutrition, allergy work or other techniques which immediately and directly affect the physical systems. Sometimes psychological problems such as irritability and tension are there largely because of mineral imbalances in the body, and the focus needs to be on the physical rather than the psychological to achieve a lasting solution to the problem. Health kinesiology recognizes that everyone is unique. The imbalances, triggers and stresses that cause eczema are likely to be different from person to person. Fortunately, the use of muscle testing means that the kinesiologist has a fast and reliable way to access this information, which is unique to each person.

Why Do People Consult A Health Kinesiologist?

They may be physically ill and want some help with their problems. Health kinesiologists have successfully treated people with a wide range of physical problems. Clients may have been through a whole range of medical tests and have no diagnosis for their symptoms. They may be anxious to reduce their dependence on drugs. They may be emotionally distressed and want help with depression, anxiety, panic attacks, lack of self-confidence, etc. An athlete may be seeking to enhance performance. A parent may be worried about a child's poor school report. A manager may be stressed by his or her workload. An accident victim suffering pain and emotional trauma, or a person who cannot see the way forward may follow up a recommendation and consult the nearest HK practitioner. People from all walks of life find an answer within health kinesiology for their needs. They respond to a system that respects the body's own inner knowledge about itself and its problems.

HK And Muscle Testing

Health kinesiology uses muscle testing to access the body's own knowledge of its needs by asking verbal questions and getting yes/no answers according to the muscle response. If the muscle is able to resist the pressure from the practitioner's hand, this means a 'yes' to the verbal question the practitioner has just asked. If the muscle weakens, this means the answer is 'no'.

The practitioner cannot ask open-ended questions (such as 'What do I do?'), because the energy system only has the on/off or yes/no response available. The practitioner must ask questions where there are only two possible responses: yes and no. Examples of these sort of questions are:

- Does the client need to drink more water?
- Do we next do procedure X?
- Is everything correct so far?

Energy imbalances can be corrected by finding a way of triggering a key stress to make the system go out of balance, then simply touching the correct combination of points to rebalance the system. Anything that causes a disturbance can be addressed. It may be something emotional or intellectual, or an allergen, a toxin, a micro-organism, a sensory input, an electromagnetic frequency, a geopathic or psychic energy: the possibilities are endless.

Muscle testing is also used to establish any beneficial adjustments to diet or a need for nutritional supplements. Advantageous changes in work, rest, sleep, play, or exercise can be found through muscle testing. The use of herbal or energy remedies (such as essences, essential oils and homeopathic remedies) can be evaluated. Health kinesiology is structured so that the practitioner can quickly home in on exactly what is needed.

Accurate Questioning

Health kinesiology, unlike many of the other kinesiology systems, relies extensively on verbal questioning. This is one of the fastest and most reliable ways to access the body's inner wisdom. It demands a high level of skill on the part of the practitioner: the precision with which questions are asked is vitally important.

Many years ago one of my sons was sent home from school with what appeared to be flu. Later that day I started to suffer with similar symptoms, and I tested whether or not I had the flu. The answer was 'no'. As the day wore on it became very clear to me that I did have flu. I was exasperated with the muscle testing because I **knew** I had flu regardless of what my body thought. The next day there was a headline in the newspaper saying that an epidemic of flu and flu-like illnesses was sweeping Britain. So, I asked my body if I had a flu-like illness and the answer was that I did. My energy system was obviously readily able to distinguish between flu and a flu-like illness, even if my intellect were not.

This sort of response is similar to that experienced with computers, which also operate on a binary system of on/off. The commonly repeated saying: 'Garbage in, garbage out' applies to verbal muscle testing just as much as to communicating with computers. When clients first experience muscle testing they usually assume that the skill is in the muscle testing itself, whereas in fact it is in the precision of the verbal questioning and the clarity of the concepts that are used.

What About The Placebo Effect?

Many HK practitioners have worked with people who are mentally handicapped to the extent that they could have no conscious concept of what was happening to them, and still the client improved. Working with babies and animals also suggests that the success of health kinesiology cannot simply be attributed to faith or the placebo effect. The client does not need to believe that the treatment will work.

> Some time ago a man came to see me. I started to take the case history and asked him what was wrong. He told me that he had severe arthritis in his knees, and then he added that he did not believe I would be able to help him. I was taken aback and asked him why he had come to see me, if he did not believe I could help him. He explained that both his wife and a next-door neighbour were clients of mine and they were always 'nagging' him to come and see me. He told me that it was worth spending the money in order to stop them nagging. I thanked him for being so honest and carried on with the session. Although he was only in his thirties, the arthritis had become so painful that he had given up his own very successful business and was now working for someone else part time. By the time he returned for his third appointment he had got himself a new job working full time for a company almost one hundred miles away. In his first month with them he had driven almost four thousand miles in his non-automatic car. He had started as a sceptic but was now totally convinced that what I had done had worked. He said that there was no way he could have driven that car for that many miles without the help of health kinesiology.

Small babies are a good example of how kinesiology is not simply based on the placebo effect.

> One of the youngest clients I ever had was a baby who was six weeks old and was failing to thrive. In fact, she was losing weight because she was sick every time she was fed. Different feeds had been tried but without any success. The baby was brought to see me. She slept through the whole session, as I used her mother as a surrogate for testing (see page 24). I established that she was allergic to the tap water that was used to mix the feed. This problem was quickly solved; the baby stopped being sick and started to gain weight much to everyone's relief. This dramatic result can hardly be attributed to the placebo effect.

Who Or What Is Responding To The Questioning?

We do not have a complete answer to this, and some kinesiologists would not agree with my views. I believe that part of the answer lies in the homeostatic mechanism of the body, which monitors body processes and adjusts hormone levels, etc, in an attempt to maintain an optimum environment. The body may not process information in terms of medical parameters, such as blood pressure being 180/110, but it does have a sense that it is too high and attempts, through various physiological mechanisms, to rectify this. Muscle testing, in part, accesses this homeostatic knowledge of the body.

But the information the health kinesiologist receives clearly goes beyond this knowledge of physiological processes. It seems to be accessing some inner wisdom. I do not know what this inner wisdom is, but I do know that if we use muscle testing wisely and rigorously we can achieve some outstanding results. For the sake of convenience health kinesiologists say that they are talking to 'the body' or 'the energy system'.

Muscle testing undoubtedly allows therapists to go beyond their intellectual understanding of the subject. Over the years I have occasionally had male clients who, according to muscle testing, needed work doing on relaxin. I was always mystified and slightly embarrassed by this, because relaxin is the hormone that relaxes the pelvis and the cervix towards the end of pregnancy. This did not seem relevant to male clients! Nevertheless, I honoured what the body told me usually with very good results. It was only recently that I read that relaxin has a role to play in maintaining the stability of the joints in men as well as women.

Many years ago muscle testing showed me that many eczema sufferers were allergic to the house dust mite. When I spoke to doctors about this, they regarded it as a bizarre idea. Now this concept is part of mainstream medical thinking about eczema. This information was initially beyond my conscious understanding and certainly beyond that of the client, but still the body's inner wisdom was able to produce the solution.

Sometimes clients' initial response to muscle testing is that the practitioner is pressing harder to make the muscle give way: they are incredulous about what is happening and this is the only reason they can find to explain the changing muscle response. It can be quite difficult to convince them that this is not the case.

Occasionally, clients try to influence the results by letting their arm give way or trying extra hard to hold it in place. One small child was determined to be allergic to cabbage, and a woman was convinced that her husband was responsible for her problems. The skilled therapist will recognize this and make allowances in the testing.

The analysis and work done is based on a combination of the body's inner wisdom and the therapist's intention, experience and knowledge. This pooling of information should allow the very best programme of work to be devised for the client. Sometimes, however, limitations in the practitioner's knowledge and assumptions that are unwittingly made influence the testing. In these circumstances less than ideal results may be obtained. No HK practitioner is one hundred per cent successful at all times, but practitioners work to ensure that they are constantly extending their knowledge and understanding of health kinesiology and the body's energy system.

Each Practitioner's Unique Perspective

Practitioners develop their own way of interpreting and working with the system. This reflects the practitioner's own strengths and interests and allows for the rich diversity that is possible with health kinesiology.

An analogy of a plate of cakes can make this clearer. When asked to choose the cake they want, one person might ask for the chocolate cake, another for the cake with the cream in the middle and another for the one with the nut on top. They could all be talking about the same cake: a chocolate cake with cream in the middle and a nut on top. Because of their own individual preferences, each person labels it in a different way. So it is with health kinesiology. There are usually numerous different ways of resolving a problem at an energy level.

Working At A Deep Level

Health kinesiologists prefer wherever possible to work at a deep level. This involves not just fixing immediate problems, but also helping clients to function more effectively in their lives. If only superficial problems are helped, people will constantly need to come back for support and new work for similar problems. This is necessary for some people where damage to the physical body is so severe it cannot be fully restored to health.

Health kinesiology practitioners are not interested in helping people re-arrange the furniture so that their lives are more comfortable. We are there to do a thorough spring clean so that the person can become the person they were designed to be. This can sound rather alarming to a new client, but health kinesiology is very gentle and respectful of the client's needs. Because the work done is always established through muscle testing, clients are not forced to address things they are not ready for.

HK is deeply self-empowering. In fact, clients sometimes do not attribute improvements to the health kinesiology work. They feel that they made the decisions themselves. This is true, but the health kinesiology work probably helped to remove enough stress so that the client could see what was needed. One client told me that she had 'opened the door herself', but that I had helped her through HK to reach the doorknob to do this.

"My odd days of feeling well became every day feeling well"

For the last eight months or so I have been experiencing this therapy with Sonia on a regular basis. I have to say I do not fully understand how it works as it is not a simple combination of tools and their application. However, I understand as much as I need to know to take part. The idea of the "body" doing the talking at first seemed strange but I enjoyed relaxing and leaving the work to my body and Sonia. The interesting thing is that something negative I may have experienced as far back as infancy (and before) has affected the efficiency of my body, but without this therapy I would not have made this connection. As a result I have come to live with an ineffectual body which in turn affects the way I think and behave. Seeing the improvement in my body has been a great thrill. I am sure there is still a lot that can be done to improve my body, but the benefits I already feel have encouraged a more positive outlook on life in general.

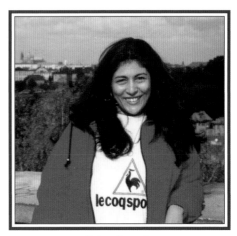

Erica Karpaiya

Approximately one month ago, I began to notice that my odd days of feeling well became every day feeling well and this happened quite suddenly following my last session with Sonia. My weight usually fluctuates from day to day, but I have remained the same weight for three weeks. I also noticed I don't wake up feeling tired and I still have some energy in the evenings.

So I started to pay more attention to feeling good and took risks with making decisions I had wanted to make for some time. I was increasingly unhappy about my job and decided on the spur of the moment to apply for another job – I got the job! My domestic arrangements caused a lot of stress. Again quite suddenly I felt able to tackle this with confidence and make decisions that would improve the situation for me. It worked!

I believe the way I feel now is directly related to the kinesiology I have been having. I now feel encouraged to attempt the exercise I know I need to do; encouraged to improve my diet and generally retake control of my body, as if someone has given me a head start with a boost of confidence and energy.

Client *Erica Karpaiya* and Practitioner *Sonia Desiderio*

One of the most precious moments in my relationship with clients is when they say that as a result of the HK they feel at peace with themselves. This is sometimes far more important to them than the original complaint they first came with. A client said to me when she came for her second appointment: "This sounds really crazy, but I feel really happy even though my acne is the same - somehow it doesn't seem so important now I feel so good inside." Another client said: "For the first time in my life, I feel really at peace with myself – oh, and by the way, my eczema has gone."

HK is a truly holistic therapy - it works with the whole person, healing them deep inside. The process is respectful and gentle, empowering the client rather than the therapist.

A Simple But Powerful System

Many people seem to need to make things unnecessarily complicated. They feel life is designed to be a struggle and filled with hardship. They believe that the only things worth having are things for which they struggle. Many people believe that they only learn through pain and distress, that they are unworthy of happiness or even that happiness would be boring and tedious. All of these feelings stimulate their need to believe also that their healing is complicated and difficult. It has to be expensive and high tech, or else demand major sacrifices and changes in their lifestyle. This is not so: health kinesiology is a powerful, relatively inexpensive therapy offering hope and healing to many people.

3: What Happens In A Health Kinesiology Session?

To an uninformed onlooker what happens in a health kinesiology session may seem beyond belief. Because many of the techniques and procedures used interact with the body's subtle energy system rather than the physical body, they often appear bizarre and even laughable. It is not uncommon for a client to come back for a second appointment saying that they left the first session feeling that they had totally wasted their money, but that the improvement in their health and sense of well-being speaks for itself. Others respond immediately to muscle testing, recognizing and becoming excited by the idea that here is a powerful way to access the person's own inner knowledge and understanding about what is needed. They appreciate that they are treated as an individual and not just offered a standard treatment.

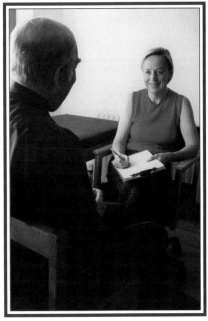

Taking the case history

When a client consults a health kinesiologist for the first time, they should find that a few moments are spent putting them at their ease. Many clients are initially nervous, uncertain that this rather bizarre-sounding therapy can help them, so usually the therapist will begin by explaining what they can expect from a session.

A medical history is taken and questions are also asked about emotional trauma, accidents, operations and any major illnesses that the person may have suffered in the past. Many practitioners will also ask about the client's goals and ambitions. This is because the practitioner is not just interested in removing ill health but in helping the client achieve what they want in life.

Then the client usually lies on a treatment couch. Some clients are worried that they might have to remove their clothes, but this is not necessary. It is also possible to work with the client standing or sitting, if this is easier for them. For example, someone who has severe back pain or is crippled with arthritis may not be able to lie comfortably on the couch.

Sometimes, when I am working with a small child and parent, we all sit on the floor within easy reach of a lot of toys. This helps to occupy the child so that they will remain relatively still.

Many clients are apprehensive about the forthcoming session, because they are unsure what to expect. They are relieved to find that the treatment is usually very gentle; some clients will even fall asleep. They will often remark afterwards on how relaxed they feel.

Surrogate Testing

Some clients are difficult to muscle test. Those who are extremely ill, elderly or frail may physically not be strong enough to hold their arm in the required position. Severely mentally handicapped people, babies, young children and animals will not have the understanding to do what is required. Yet it is possible to help even these people through the phenomenon of surrogate testing. Anyone can be used as a surrogate,

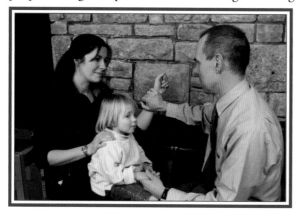

Surrogate testing

but it is often convenient to use a close relative. The surrogate and the actual client need to be touching. In this way it is possible to energy balance the client by muscle testing the surrogate. The practitioner has to have a clear intent to ask about the energy system of the client, even though the arm muscles of a different person are being used. This procedure usually works remarkably well.

Stuart Miller, an HK practitioner in Devon, used surrogate testing to help a two-year-old child, who had bright red cheeks with dry scaly skin. She was scratching her cheeks, which made it worse. She also had a spotty rash on her trunk. Stuart used the child's mother as a surrogate - they all sat on the floor. While the child played, Stuart tested her through the mother. Among other things, Stuart found and corrected an allergy for celery – the child's mother commented that she used a lot of celery in cooking. About a month later Stuart saw the child again: her cheeks had cleared, but the rash on the trunk was still causing her mother some concern. Again using the child's mother as a surrogate, Stuart carried out more HK procedures. The mother wrote to Stuart later to say that the rash cleared up soon after the session and had not returned.

Self-Testing

Sometimes, rather than testing the client's muscles, practitioners will use themselves as a surrogate, testing a muscle of their own, usually a finger. This can be much faster than testing the client's muscles. It is also used if, for some reason, the client cannot be tested directly and there is not a suitable surrogate available.

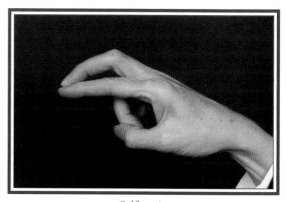

Self-testing

"He was like a different child"

Tom, aged two, was brought to see me because he'd had really bad eczema since he was two months old. He was allergic to wheat, eggs, soya and milk. He was on an extremely limited diet and on quite a lot of medication. I worked through the mother using her as a surrogate. Tom played the whole time but seemed quite happy for me to work on him and hold points or put cosbats on him. He began to improve straight away, but the improvement was erratic to begin with. The first issue was *My Eczema*. This included an SET and I also had to do some work on the geopathic stress of his house. Then we did another issue: *Exuding An Irritated Sign*, which included psychological work on being irritated. There were two more issues: *Fear That I Will Never Have Peace In My Life* and then *Strengthening My Ability To Heal Myself*. Two months later he had improved considerably. Next we did an SET on a non-wheat flour mix and specialist nutritional supplement he was taking. He continued to steadily improve. His skin stopped flaking; he was less irritable; his moods became much better, but he was still very sleepless. So I worked directly on his sleep and he started to sleep better. Then we had a couple more sessions, and I worked directly on the foods he was allergic to. I did allergy corrections for soya and milk, and then tolerance for wheat, soya, milk and eggs. Six months later his mum told me that he was like a different child: he was now a normal happy three-year old.

Client *Tom* and Practitioner *Tessa Gaynn*

The Initial Balance

The subtle energy system needs to be in balance to ensure accurate answers to the verbal questions that are central to the HK approach. At the beginning of a session most clients are not in balance. Stress in all its forms causes the energy system to become unbalanced and some people then stay out of balance. Fortunately it is usually rela-tively easy to put the energy system back into balance for the session. Most people find this a very relaxing process and some people notice physical sensations, such as tingling or warmth, while this is happening. This whole procedure will often take less than ten minutes.

The practitioner will commonly use either a muscle in the shoulder (the anterior deltoid) or one in the forearm (the brachioradialis) for muscle testing. These are convenient muscles, although almost any muscle in the body could be used. Gentle pressure is applied to check that the muscle is strong. The muscle is then pinched lengthwise lightly and the arm tested. The arm will give way, at least slightly, if the muscle is functioning correctly. This test is checking out a physiological response of the muscle: pinching the muscle produces an automatic response – the muscle relaxes to avoid injury. Clients are always surprised by this simple method of changing a muscle's state.

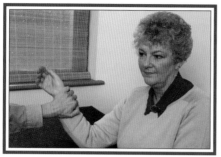

Muscle testing the brachioradialis – this can be done with the client sitting or lying down

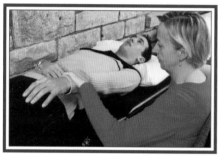

Muscle testing anterior deltoid – this can be done with client lying down, sitting or standing

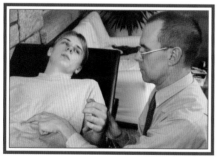

Checking test points around the navel

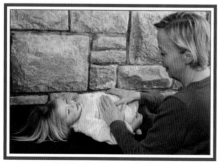

Holding points to balance the acupuncture energy system

If neither of these muscles tests strong initially, the practitioner will test other muscles until one is found that gives a strong response initially and then weakens on pinching. This is referred to as the indicator muscle. This muscle can then be used to establish whether or not the energy system is balanced and, if not, what to do about it. To do this, the practitioner gently touches one or more test points on the body and tests the arm again. If the arm gives way even slightly when this is done, this indicates that the acupuncture energy system is out of balance.

The practitioner brings the client's energy system back into balance by holding specific points on the body. This initial balancing procedure is extremely important because, if the acupuncture energy is unbalanced, the practitioner may not be able to get reliable answers to the questions they wish to ask the energy system.

When the energy system seems to be balanced, three simple checks are carried out to confirm this:

- A verbal confirmation - 'yes'/'no'.

- A confirmation using a pinch test.

- A confirmation using a magnet.

These three different tests check on different aspects of balance. If any of these tests do not confirm the energy balance, the practitioner will again hold acupuncture points and then re-do all three checks.

The Verbal Test

This involves the client saying 'yes', and their arm being tested while a hand is placed over the navel. It does not matter whether it is the hand of the practitioner or the client that is put over the navel. The hand over the navel allows the practitioner to access information on the whole of the energy system and not just information about the meridian related to the muscle that is being tested.

If the person is balanced, the arm will stay strong or locked, and the practitioner will then ask the client to say 'no' and test again. This time the arm should go down or at least become spongy if the person is balanced.

The Pinch Test

This involves pinching the middle of a muscle other than the one the practitioner is testing. Usually the quadriceps, a large muscle on the front of the thigh is used. The practitioner pinches the muscle and then immediately tests the arm muscle while a hand is once again placed over the navel. If the person is balanced, the arm will test weak. This is at first sight a rather surprising response: one muscle is pinched and another muscle switches off. This occurs because the pinch convinces the leg muscle that it is too contracted and so the muscle automatically relaxes in order to avoid over-strain and injury. The hand over the navel allows this response to be fed through to the arm muscle that is being tested.

The Magnet Test

A small magnet is used for this test. The south-seeking pole of the magnet is placed on the client's body, usually on the thigh. The practitioner then tests the arm muscle, while another hand is over the navel. If the person's energy system is balanced, the arm will test strong. When the magnet is turned over, so that the north-seeking pole is on the body, the muscle should test weak. Again the hand over the navel is allowing the response of one muscle to be mirrored in the response of another.

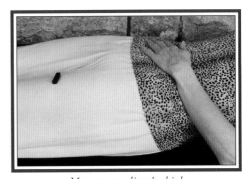

Magnet on client's thigh

The Thymus Tap

Sometimes the practitioner will use the thymus tap as a quick way of balancing the energy system. Either the practitioner or the client taps on the client's chest, in an anti-clockwise circle for about thirty seconds. This balancing tap may not be as long lasting as the initial balance and it does not work at all for some people. The three confirmatory tests are still carried out. The thymus tap can also be used between treatments by clients to help themselves stay in balance.

Talking To The Body

When the client's energy system is in balance. A 'no' response will have a similar effect to an energy disturbance, that is, it will weaken a muscle. So if the practitioner asks a question, and the client's 'body' believes the answer to be 'no', a muscle will test weak. In this way the practitioner can hold a 'conversation' with the client's body (or energy system).

Energy Permission

Once the energy system is balanced, the therapist asks the first question, which is always for energy permission to begin work. The person's conscious mind has given permission, but occasionally there is a good reason why energy work would not be appropriate, even though the client may not be consciously aware of this.

This is an extremely important part of the way in which a health kinesiologist works. The practitioner does not proceed unless he gets this energy permission. The practitioner works in a way that is respectful of the client: the client has given conscious permission by coming to see the practitioner, but the practitioner also wants to establish energy permission for the work.

If the practitioner does not get energy permission, it is sometimes possible to establish through muscle testing the exact reason for the refusal and then establish when the work can proceed. The most common reason for not getting energy permission is that the client has recently visited another type of therapist. For example, the client may have recently been given a homeopathic remedy or had a shiatsu treatment and sometimes, but not always, it is just not appropriate to introduce even more changes, however beneficial they are in principal.

To establish energy permission the therapist says:

- Do we have energy permission to work together now?

  The answer to this is usually 'yes'.

If the answer to the first question is 'yes', the practitioner then asks another question:

- Is there any reason why we should not work together now?

  Usually the answer to this is 'no'.

If the practitioner gets a 'yes' response to this second question it usually means that some minor changes need to occur before the session can proceed. The exact changes are identified through muscle testing. Common ones include giving the client a drink of water, making the client more comfortable in some way or explaining in more detail exactly what is going to happen.

> A new client came to see me, and initially I did not obtain energy permission to work unless I agreed that there were certain areas we would not touch on. The client made no comment about this. When I saw his sister a few days later for her appointment, she told me that he had told her what had happened. His wife also told her that just before his appointment he was listing all the things he was not prepared to talk to me about.

Sometimes the reason for the initial refusal relates to the practitioner rather than the client.

On one occasion I got 'yes' in answer to the second question and through muscle testing we established that I had to do something. Before the client had arrived I had made some soup (my office is an annex of my house). Once I started the session with the client I began to fret that I had not turned the soup off before I started work. I had to go and check the cooker. This was a reasonable instruction because I was hardly likely to do my best work while wondering if my house was about to burn down!

Usually, though, the client's energy system does give permission for the work to take place.

Once energy permission has been granted the same system is used throughout the session: verbal questions are asked, light pressure is applied to the arm, and the response is translated into a 'yes' or a 'no'

How Does The HK Practitioner Decide What To Do?

One of the fundamental differences between health kinesiology and many other therapies, including many other kinesiologies, is that there are no set procedures for particular problems. For example, for one person with chronic fatigue syndrome the practitioner might find they are mainly working to improve the client's ability to cope with electromagnetic pollution; with another the work might centre on allergies and psychological issues; for another powerful detoxification procedures for viruses and heavy metals might be what is needed, and sometimes a combination of all of these might be appropriate. Sometimes the choices that the body makes show the practitioner clearly how the body sees the origin of the illness, but sometimes it does not make any sense in rational terms. At this point the practitioner and client have to trust that the body's inner wisdom knows what is needed. Even two members of the same family with the same symptoms will probably receive completely different treatment. This is part of what makes HK such an intriguing and sensitive therapy: it truly respects the individual and treats him or her as unique.

The Health Kinesiology Menu

As the symptom does not dictate the treatment, the HK practitioner has to have some way of establishing what to do. There are two important decisions to be made:

- How to focus the work.
- What techniques and procedures to use.

Health kinesiology recognizes that the client's conscious understanding of what is paramount may not be correct and within HK there are protocols to establish this.

A young lady went to see Rob Adams, a practitioner based in Chester. She had chronic fatigue syndrome (ME), but her body would not give him permission to work on it in the first session, so Rob asked her if she had another problem. She said she had to go to the dentist the following Tuesday. This is what her body wanted treating first, so Rob did this. The client impressed the dentist with her calmness.

There are many different techniques and procedures at an HK practitioner's disposal, and the therapist uses muscle testing to determine, firstly, how to focus the work, and, secondly, what specific techniques and procedures to use. HK has developed an extensive range of techniques and the basic building blocks are put together in many different ways to produce a limitless number of options, so that the treatment fits the individual. Health kinesiology does not require that round pegs be fitted into square holes: the treatment is altered and adapted to the exact 'shape' of the client's needs.

This range of options is referred to as the health kinesiology menu. It means that a whole range of possibilities can be offered to the energy system, so that the treatment can be uniquely programmed to that individual.

Incorporating Other Therapies

Some HK practitioners are also skilled in other therapies, such as reflexology or reiki or Bowen therapy. The practitioner will include these possibilities in the options that are offered to the energy system. These therapies can then be included in the session if indicated by testing.

Diverse Possibilities

Clients are often amazed at the diversity of things that happen during a typical HK session. One moment they may have to think a specific thought, and then they may have to put their hands in specific positions on their body. On another occasion they may find that small vials, crystals or magnets are placed on the body. Much of the time the practitioner will also be holding points or placing multi-coloured glass tubes on the body. A client once said to me that he found the sessions so fascinating that he would be tempted to come and see me even if he weren't getting better. Each technique and procedure is established precisely through muscle testing. On its completion the practitioner will also check, again using muscle testing, that everything has happened correctly.

"No needles and no nasty mixtures!!"

A ganglion had appeared on my left hand wrist. It was very painful so I thought I would go to the doctors. After one visit, the doctor told me what it was and with time, my ganglion would start to go away, but it didn't. About two months later I went to the doctors for a second time. This time the doctor booked me an appointment with the orthopaedic surgeon. I really didn't want to undergo an operation so I looked for an alternative way for it to be removed. I tried alternative medicine.

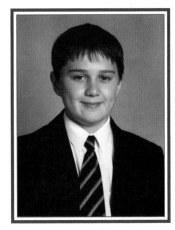

Jamie Mallinson

When I went to my first session, I really didn't know what to expect. I thought of needles being prodded into me, and taking horrid potions. It was neither. All that happened was Sandra put my body into balance, using a magnet then asking my body questions using my arm. No needles and no nasty mixtures!! She made me put two or three test tubes on my navel, then, with my finger, to touch the centre of my ganglion. After a couple of minutes I felt a strange tingling sensation in my ganglion. It was energy entering the lump!

At the end of the session, she told me to wear a gizmo [see glossary], when I went to sleep. By the morning, I looked at my ganglion and it was far less painful and it had gone all squishy around the edges! After a few days, the lump went down a lot. About a month later, it went completely. It has never come back, and the area where it was doesn't hurt at all.

Alternative medicine is a great option to choose to get rid of just about anything!!

Client *Jamie Mallinson* (age 13) and Practitioner *Sandra Shackleton*

How Does The Practitioner Know When A Procedure Is Completed?

Clients are often intrigued that the practitioner will spend varying amounts of time on each procedure, so a common question is: "How do you know when it is time to move on?"

Most practitioners have their own special signal that things have been completed. The most common signal is yawning, although others include changes in the eye blinking rate and change in the tension of the diaphragm. Some practitioners will feel gentle pulsing in the client's body where they are touching the client. When the practitioner believes that a procedure is complete, this is checked by muscle testing.

Sometimes the client will sigh or open their eyes (if they were closed) when the procedure is completed. Clients may also be consciously aware that the procedure is complete, and say: "I think it is done now."

How Does The Client Feel During The Session?

An HK session is usually an extremely gentle process and people often fall asleep during it. Some clients do cry or experience emotional release. Others experience physical symptoms during treatment, e.g. trembling, muscle spasm, heat, tingling, heaviness, yawning or strange tummy noises. This does not seem to indicate how effective the work will be, but it is helpful for clients to have this internal validation that something is going on.

Often the client will be surprised at what is found and say, for example: "Sometimes I get a pain in the exact place where you placed the magnet, but I didn't tell you because I thought it wasn't important". Clients are often amazed when muscle testing produces information that the client knows to be correct, but has not told the practitioner.

Some years ago I was recording an interview for a radio programme. The interviewer told me that he had allergy problems and wanted to base the interview around what I would do to fix this. I got him balanced, started testing and found that his energy system wanted a detoxification for tranquillisers as the first part of the treatment. I asked him if he had ever taken tranquillisers. He immediately switched off his recording machine and told me that some years previously he had been an in-patient in a psychiatric hospital. His current employer did not know about this. He was amazed at what I had found and very relieved that the programme was not going out live.

Christine Fowler, a practitioner in the north east of England, was testing out some nutrition information for a client. Christine established through the muscle testing that the client should stop working at lunchtime, sit down in a quiet place and eat her food. The client was taken aback, because she had not told Christine that she normally ate 'on the hoof' at lunchtime.

Homework

When all the session work is completed the practitioner will muscle test if there is anything else to do. This includes any work that clients need to do for themselves. Homework might include following a precise exercise programme, following a specific schedule for rest and sleep, or taking nutritional supplements. The client might need to take a homeopathic remedy or flower essences.

The End Of The Session

Certain questions are asked before the practitioner stops working on the client. Two of the most important ones are:

- Do we have energy permission to stop?

- Is there any reason why we should not stop?

These questions are vitally important because they help to safeguard the work that has been done. If the practitioner has omitted something important, the energy system will not give the practitioner permission to stop.

At the end of the session the practitioner may ask through muscle testing:

- Is there any more work to schedule?

Sometimes the practitioner does not need to specifically to ask this question, because it has become clear earlier in the session that a programme of work is necessary, which will take more than a single session.

If further work is needed, the practitioner will want to know when the next session should be. The practitioner once again will ask questions using muscle testing to establish the answer. This part of the session always seems to intrigue new clients. Yet it makes sense that there may be restrictions on when the next lot of work can take place. Often the body needs time to process the work done in a session: the changes happen instantly at a certain energy level, but then have to be processed through to the physical body, and emotional and psychological changes may need to take place before the next session.

Another frequent question at the end of a session is:

- Is there anything we need to know about the next session?

This is a very useful question because the client may need to bring something specific for allergy testing, for example.

How Long Before The Client Notices An Improvement?

Many practitioners will also muscle test to see what benefit the client can expect to see before the next appointment. Sometimes there will be no specific benefit, because the work needs to be processed, and the healing needs to occur over a longer period of time. The work may be of a preliminary nature, and so the client will not be aware of any positive benefit. Sometimes the client will notice a gradual improvement over the next few weeks and months. Sometimes nothing will appear to happen, and then suddenly one day there will be a dramatic improvement.

Some clients, however, notice an immediate, dramatic benefit from the treatment.

One client got off the couch and said to me: "I didn't feel anything." I explained that some clients do not experience anything while they are lying on the couch but that does not mean that they will not get better. She said: "No, I didn't mean that. What I meant was that I experienced no pain when I got off the couch." She had had a hip replacement operation seven years earlier and told me, when I was taking the case history, that she had simply changed one constant pain (from her damaged hip) for another constant pain (the artificial hip). She was extremely surprised and excited that she had been able to get off the couch without experiencing any pain.

What Will The Improvement Be?

Health kinesiologists do not predict the future, but they can use muscle testing to establish the likely outcome of the session. Prediction involves being able to see into the future, whereas the HK practitioner uses muscle testing to project what will happen if everything occurs as expected.

So the practitioner can ask questions such as:

- Will the client notice any improvements in their existing symptoms as a result of the treatment?

- Will the client notice any mental benefits (e.g. increased concentration, better memory) as a result of the treatment?

- Will the client have more energy as a result of the treatment?

- Will the client feel more confident as a result of the treatment?

These questions allow the therapist to estimate when the person will be well and how they will experience the benefit. This is a difficult skill to acquire, and it also does not take into account circumstances that may change which the therapist cannot foresee.

One client produced results that differed from my projection on two separate occasions. She was a professional climber and had come to see me because of her injured back. She had been injured in a fall over a year before and had not been able to climb since. She had tried many different forms of therapy, none of which had worked. Some had even made the problem worse. At the end of the first session I established through muscle testing that she would see no improvement before the next session and told her this. She came back for her next session and told me that her back was much better - much to my surprise. During the analysis in the first session I had discovered that she was allergic to the contraceptive pill that she was taking. Her body was busy minimizing her reaction to the pill to the extent that she was unaware that she had a problem with it. Because of this, it had limited resources to heal the back. Through testing I established that we could not do anything about the allergy to the pill for several sessions. I explained this to her, but she said that she had to take the pill, because all the alternatives were unacceptable and she was determined not to become pregnant. She had, however, gone home and decided not to take the pill, and so her body had started the healing process. The assessment about the lack of improvement had been based on the assumption that she was going to continue taking the contraceptive pill between sessions.

At the end of the second session I tested that her back would continue to improve. She came back for the third session and told me that she was much worse again. I immediately asked her if she had started taking the contraceptive pill again, and she assured me that she had not. I was disappointed that she had not continued to improve and wondered if I had made a mistake. Half way through the session she told me that she had been feeling so well that she had been climbing and had fallen again. So once again the assessment at the end of the second session was probably correct, but it did not take into account that she would start climbing again and have another fall.

The Healing Process

Sometimes the client will feel worse either during the session or in the subsequent few days. This is common to many therapies and is usually referred to as a healing crisis, but Jimmy Scott prefers to refer to it as a healing process. He argues that the word crisis implies something negative whereas what is happening is in fact something very positive. I often liken it to spring-cleaning. In the process of healing itself the energy system may have to clear out a lot of debris. This can result in existing symptoms becoming worse, or the emergence of flu- or cold-type symptoms, headaches, strange bowel movements and rancid-smelling sweat.

Maggie Dewis, a practitioner based near Colchester, helped a three-year-old boy. He had been born to a fifteen-year-old mother who was in foster care. The mother did not accept that she was pregnant until the baby was almost due. He was born four weeks early. The mother gave him up at birth, and he was adopted when he was almost three months old. As he grew older those involved became concerned about his development. He saw a string of specialists – a speech therapist, a psychologist, a paediatrician and a special needs health visitor. There was concern that the child had attention deficit disorder or even a personality disorder. At the end of the first session Maggie warned the parents that there would be a reaction to the treatment in seven days. The child's mother said later: "The reaction was profound: ... (he) was impossible, difficult and unhappy for a whole weekend. We could not do a thing with him!" After that weekend he settled down and the parents and the nursery teachers noticed a general improvement. Two months later Maggie saw him again. This time his mother commented: "Since this treatment ... (he) has 'come on' in leaps and bounds. He is more confident and outgoing, enjoys socialising with everybody and is now communicating in all the right ways."

As the healing process can mean that the client appears to be worse after a session, it is important for the practitioner to be able to distinguish between a healthy healing process, and a treatment that has not worked. In general this is not difficult to do. If it is a healing process the client will, when questioned, often be able to identify some way in which the current situation is different from the normal symptoms. So, for example, the client might say that he normally loses his sense of smell when his sinuses are bad, but this time he has not, or that he is actually feeling cheerful and energetic, even though the pain is very bad. In addition, the healing process does not usually last longer than about five days. If the exacerbation of symptoms goes on beyond this, the practitioner will usually have the client back, so that they can check through muscle testing what is going on.

"Everything had disappeared."

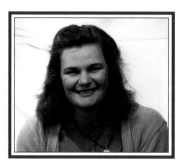

Martine Fontaine

Mathieu, a young boy of eleven, was born with eczema all over his body. Now he just has some in the bends of his knees and elbows. His skin is like a molehill field with lots of scars because of the scratching.

For the first session we were only allowed to do one group of BBEIs (see chapter 6). I could see some scepticism rising in his mother's eyes, but she did not say anything. When they came for the second session she was satisfied because everything had disappeared. In this session we are only allowed to do one group of corrections because Mathieu is going on holiday to Italy.

After his holiday we do an SET (see chapter 9). The eczema starts again more present than ever. I reassured the mother and tested that it will be approximately three weeks, then it will disappear again. And that is what happened!

Client *Mathieu Paternostre* and Practitioner *Martine Fontaine* (Belgium)

Length Of Appointments

In general, appointments last one to one and a half hours, but occasionally muscle testing will demand longer or shorter sessions.

A client with severe vertigo came to see me. He needed several sessions spread over several months. Each lasted about ten minutes. This disjointed treatment schedule, found through muscle testing, was dictated by his energy system. It wanted a small change made, and then time to absorb and process it before the next change. Fortunately the client was very patient. He came to see me the required number of times and his vertigo disappeared completely.

How Many Sessions Are Needed?

Prospective clients often ask: "How many sessions will I need?" There is no standard answer: it depends entirely on the individual.

The number of sessions does not necessarily even relate to the severity of the problem, nor does it relate to the length of time that the client has had the symptoms. I have had clients with a small patch of eczema who have needed five or six sessions to see the benefit, and I have also had some truly miraculous results for severe or long-standing problems in the space of one or two sessions. The HK practitioner has to be guided by the muscle testing and proceed at the correct pace for the individual client.

A Simple But Powerful System

When people first experience health kinesiology they are often amazed at how little appears to happen in a session. People will often say: "It can't be that simple", or "Is that it?" Healing is often very simple if only we do the right thing. Miraculous results do happen, even with people who have had long-standing problems. Whatever is needed is tailored specifically to the individual and the individual's deep inner knowledge of how to achieve health and harmony.

"I'm now looking forward to more sessions and more results."

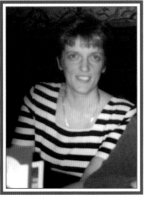

Janice Lake

I've always been interested in alternative therapies but had never heard of health kinesiology until a colleague told me about it. I obtained a leaflet and after reading it I thought that it might be able to help me, so I booked an appointment.

I had just changed my job from one that I loved to a promotion nearer to my home, which would enable me to spend more time with my family. However, I was finding it extremely stressful and had been very much dropped in it at the deep end. With almost no training I was expected to run a busy office, co-ordinate staff and set up support systems for the department. As well as this, I was not made to feel welcome in my new position. Yes, I had more time with my family, but I was stressed, tired and my confidence was taking such a battering that I was not a nice person to be with.

At my first session, I really didn't know what to expect. Sue (my practitioner) asked me some general questions. I'm asthmatic and need to take regular medication. We talked about what I hoped to gain from the sessions. My priority was to deal with my stress, lack of confidence, tiredness and the headaches that I'd been experiencing. I found the session to be extremely relaxing and many psychological issues were brought up that were very relevant to me – Sue would have no way of knowing these beforehand.

When I've tried describing the session to friends, I find it very difficult – you have to have an open mind and relax. At the very least it was extremely relaxing.

The following weekend I felt wonderful. However, on my return to work, the stress of my job overwhelmed me again. After three sessions with Sue I decided that the job was not working out, and I made the decision to leave. Once I had come to that decision I felt much better, even though my future felt insecure. I had never been in that position before, as I had always left a job to take up another. However, I worked hard to gain employment and within two weeks had accomplished this.

Another benefit I feel is attributable to HK concerns my allergy to animals. Usually when I visit my sister who has a dog, I last about half an hour before sneezing and wheezing. On my last two visits I stayed in the same room as the dog for three hours and suffered no adverse effects. I also cleaned my daughter's rabbits when she was ill and again with no difficulty.

I'm now looking forward to more sessions and more results.

Client *Janice Lake* and Practitioner *Sue Morgan*

4: Organizing The Work

In health kinesiology we do not have specific techniques or treatment for specific symptoms or problems. Each person is treated as a unique individual, whose energy system will reveal what procedures are needed, and exactly how they should be carried out.

Once the practitioner has taken the client's case history and made sure the acupuncture system is balanced (see page 25), the practitioner then has to establish exactly how to proceed with the work and what work to do. The power of health kinesiology is that the practitioner does not have to try to work out intellectually or intuitively where the problem lies, but uses muscle testing to identify the areas to be rebalanced.

There are five recognized ways of structuring or organizing a session and the energy system will have a preference for one particular way. The five possible ways are:

- Working according to an issue named by the client – referred to as *a client specified issue* (see page 40).

- Grouping the work under an issue title identified by muscle testing – referred to as *an HK tested iss*ue (see page 42).

- Working in overall body sequence (see page 46).

- Using meridian analysis (see page 47).

- Using meta analysis (see page 47).

The practitioner establishes which of these is the appropriate way to work by offering the body the five possibilities through verbal questioning and muscle testing, and allowing the energy system to choose:

- Do we work in terms of a client specified issue?

If the practitioner got a weak response (a 'no' answer) to this, then he/she would ask about the other options:

- Do we work in terms of an HK tested issue?

If the muscle gave a strong response to working in terms of a client specified issue, the practitioner would ask about each of the problems/symptoms named by the client:

- So, do we work on Valerie's eczema?"

This questioning process continues until the exact issue is worked out. When working with a client I often have in mind the analogy of a library. I see us all as having a library of books about how to make ourselves what we are intended to be. Health kinesiology is a very useful tool for accessing this library.

Working According To An Issue Named By The Client

When a client comes for an HK session they usually have particular problems in mind. The HK practitioner tries, if possible, to address these concerns, providing the energy system gives permission. Usually the energy system is prepared to do this, because, if the imbalance within the body is sufficient to produce visible physical symptoms or conscious awareness, it is usually important enough to take priority.

When the therapist works with an issue title named by the client, **the client** is choosing 'the book'. The client tells the therapist what they want, e.g. "I want my in-growing toe nails sorted out." In this case the practitioner, using muscle testing, goes into the 'library' and finds the 'book' relating to fixing this problem for the client. The therapist 'opens the book and reads the information in it': the instructions about how to fix the client's in-growing toenails. These instructions are expressed in terms of health kinesiology techniques, nutritional requirements, other remedies, and so on. It may be necessary to fine-tune through muscle testing the exact wording for the title.

In general this approach works well, particularly with new clients. They need to be convinced of the value of health kinesiology, and fixing what they are worrying about usually does the trick. This, for them, is proof that this 'weird stuff' works. Returning clients may also want specific symptoms or problems addressed, and providing the therapist gets energy permission it is usually possible to do this.

In this situation the issue title relates directly and obviously to a symptom or a named illness. The client describes the problem, and the exact wording of the issue title is established by muscle testing. For example, if the client came with asthma then the issue title might be *Healing My Asthma* or *My Asthma Is A Nuisance*.

Sometimes the energy system is not prepared to work on the problem identified by the client. This can be for several reasons:

1.   The energy system might demand work on another symptom.

Amanda Pollard was working with Tracey Watts, and the energy system produced the issue title *My Sweating*. Amanda asked Tracey if this meant anything to her, as sweating had not been mentioned when discussing her symptoms. She told Amanda that in fact she did not sweat properly: at work her skin would feel clammy, and she would be boiling hot, but there was no sweat, so she was always putting the fan on. A month later she was already reporting that she was sweating more, and that she was feeling more energetic.

A client with very serious health problems consulted me: she was suffering from hot flushes as a side-effect of some of her medication and she came for help for this. When I asked her energy system to give me permission to work on this, it refused. Her energy system insisted that first we had to focus on her very real and justified fear of dying. When I explained this to her she was happy for us to work in this area first.

2. The energy system might want to deal with the named symptom in a bigger, seemingly unrelated issue.

    A bank manager consulted me for nail biting. He told me that he had bitten his nails for the whole of his life. Apart from looking unsightly, it was professionally very embarrassing. On testing, his body produced the issue *My Relationship With Women*. The client commented that he did not have any problems relating to women, but agreed that we should proceed with the work anyway. He returned for his second appointment approximately ten days later and said: "I still don't think I've got any problem relating to women, but I have stopped biting my nails."

3. Sometimes the energy system wants to collect an apparently disparate array of symptoms and deal with them altogether. From the point of view of the client, and even of the therapist, the symptoms seem distinct and separate, but the body itself understands that they are all linked together.

    A client consulted me about sinus problems and headaches. Through muscle testing I established that we could deal with these problems, but we had to collect the work we would do together under the issue title of *Expressing Longings*. It transpired that the client had never got over the death of her mother. The work we did was designed to help her to come to terms with her mother's death, as well as to help the physical problems. After we found the issue title she told me that her sinus problems had been worse since her mother's death.

4. The energy system might choose to work on a seemingly minor symptom that has just started rather than on a more serious and chronic problem. In this case the body seems to be taking a pragmatic view. The client has had the chronic problem for many years so an extra few weeks is neither here nor there, whereas the new symptom will escalate rapidly in the next few weeks, so it makes sense to deal with this first.

5. The energy system might ask for much more than the conscious mind is prepared to. I am constantly struck by how little improvement in health people request, particularly as they get older, presumably because they have been led to believe that deteriorating health is inevitable. Sometimes clients will not mention symptoms because they believe that nothing can be done about them. Sometimes they will mention them but say things like: "What can I expect at my age?" or " It runs in my

family, so I suppose it will just get worse". HK can be of enormous help with all kinds of conditions, including 'inherited' ones and those associated with old age. The innate wisdom of the body recognizes this and, through the muscle testing, will ask to achieve more. So an elderly client may come for help with an allergic rash and be surprised that the HK practitioner also works on their arthritis.

HK Tested Issue

HK issue titles, also referred to as priority issues, are one of the most fascinating parts of health kinesiology. Continuing with the library analogy, when practitioners are working according to HK tested issues, they are using muscle testing to find out which book should be taken down off the library shelves – **the energy system** is determining the priority work to be done. Once the book has been found, muscle testing is again used to 'read' what health kinesiology techniques are needed. The energy system demands particular wording to ensure that the problem is covered as comprehensively yet as precisely as possible.

Working like this, the practitioner is tapping into the inner wisdom of the energy system and working for the person's higher good, rather than just dealing with immediate symptoms. The energy system gathers the work together and gives it a named focus: the HK issue title. The practitioner uses systematic questioning to establish the exact title of the issue. The practitioner cannot ask the question: "What is the priority issue title?" because the muscle testing can only produce 'yes' or 'no' as an answer. So, a series of questions are asked, such as:

- Can this issue be defined in physical terms?

- Can this issue be defined in psychological terms?

- Can this issue be defined in spiritual terms?

- Are there at least three words in the issue title?

- Is the word 'my' included in the issue title?

- Are the names of any people included in the issue title?

From this systematic questioning the practitioner can usually quickly find priority issue titles whether it is *Healing My Respiratory System* or *My Relationship With Anthony* or *Finding My Spiritual Path*.

The issue title is not a diagnosis or an instruction. So, muscle testing could produce the issue title *Leaving My Husband*, but this is not an **instruction** to do so. The issue title *Being Stupid* does not mean that the client **is** stupid. The issue title is simply a way of organizing the work.

"Total relief from asthma symptoms"

Alex was fourteen when he came to see me. He is an intelligent and very active young man who is particularly keen on rowing in his school team. He had suffered from asthma since he was seven, which may have been precipitated by his parents' divorce when he was six. He caught frequent colds and chest infections and often had to spend days in bed with migraine. He had to use an asthma inhaler regularly twice a

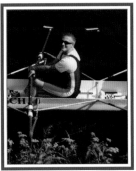 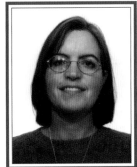

Alex Fenton   *Janice Hocking*

day, in addition to a bronchial dilator spray before any form of physical exertion. His favourite sport of rowing brought on severe pain and wheezing. I saw Alex three times over a period of five weeks, but after our first session he did not suffer any asthma attacks again and eventually was able to put his asthma drugs away in a drawer.

The first session had an issue title: *Improving My Self-Confidence*. As well as corrections, muscle testing revealed that Alex had to avoid all dairy products, wheat and tomato for a while, which meant that his favourite meal of pizza was definitely off the menu for a while. With help from his mother and advice from me, he stuck to these dietary restrictions. I am convinced that the excellent results we obtained from these sessions were greatly helped by Alex's willingness to follow my advice.

Our next issue was called *Boosting The Energy Flow To My Nervous System* and finally we did *Boosting The Energy Flow To All Parts Of My Respiratory System*. This included an SET correction with thirteen different substances, including both of his asthma drugs and a homeopathic sample of pneumonia bacteria. Although I hadn't worked directly on the migraine, this disappeared along with the asthma and to date he has not had another episode of pain or wheezing.

Fourteen weeks later I was able to do three more sessions on Alex, each time removing the allergy to one of the foods - dairy first, then wheat and finally tomato. He followed the programme I set up for gradually reintroducing these foods to his diet, and can now eat as much pizza as he likes!

Alex subsequently sent me a letter to thank me for all the help I'd given him. He wrote, "even after one session I found total relief from asthma symptoms. Ever since I have never felt better and I would recommend this treatment to anyone because it has really changed my life."

Client *Alex Fenton* and Practitioner *Janice Hocking*

Sometimes priority issue titles can be very poignant. Some years ago a client came to see me with a weak heart. The issue title we found was *Broken-Hearted*. This was particularly moving because one of her grandchildren was suffering from an unrelated heart condition and was seriously ill. My client was extremely upset about the pain and suffering of her grandchild: she was indeed broken-hearted in more ways than one. For another client *Treadmill* summed up how he felt about his life. *Cutting The Umbilical Cord* made a teenager look pensive. Another client's issue title was *There's Something Wrong With My Vision*. He immediately related this to his poor eyesight, but subsequently also related it to his restricted view of his future.

When I have found a priority issue title I sometimes want to smile:

- *The Liver Meridian Won't Do What It Should* sounded like a cry of exasperation from the energy system.

- *Being The Sickest Client* brought a chuckle from the client - one of my longest-standing clients, who sometimes rejoiced in how complicated she was.

- *My Role As A Frightened Worrier* had the client smiling at the appropriateness of it.

- *Being A Troublesome Woman* brought hoots of laughter from myself and a long-standing feisty female client.

One particularly moving example of the power of finding the priority issue occurred during a workshop. A student volunteered for the demonstration, and the priority issue came up as her relationship with a particular woman. I asked various questions through the muscle testing, such as:

- Is this a blood relative?

- Does the client still know the woman?

From the testing it became clear that the person we were seeking was not a blood relative, the student did not know if the woman was still alive and, in fact, did not even know the name of the woman.

I began to doubt my muscle testing, because it seemed unlikely that the priority issue could relate to her relationship with a woman whose name she did not know. Suddenly the student's face went white, and she said that she thought she knew who it was. I tested to see if her surmise was correct, and it was. She then explained that one of her children had been stillborn and that she had always blamed the midwife who had delivered the baby. Later in the day she told me that once we had found the priority issue title, she realised that all her subsequent relationships with everyone had been coloured by her feelings about this woman. She also said that if anyone had asked her beforehand if she had recovered from the loss of her child, she would have said 'yes'. It was only with the finding of the priority issue title that she was brought face-to-face with her own deep feelings. For her the finding of the priority issue title was in itself a powerful and healing process.

"The result of the test showed that Margaret had no thrombotic tendencies."

Twenty five years ago I had my first spontaneous thrombosis at age twenty five. I came out of hospital with a daily dosage of warfarin to take. The dose was gradually reduced and after about six months I came off it. I have been left with permanent damage to an area of my lung; fortunately my heart has not been affected.

At age thirty I began experiencing a repeat of the symptoms and was put back on warfarin. The consultant recommended that I continue the medication for the rest of my life. Although I was devastated, I decided that I would carry on with the warfarin: a small price to pay to keep me free of clots in the future until I found an alternative.

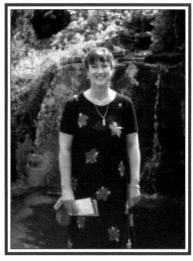

Margaret Leadbetter

Slowly my health deteriorated, probably due to a combination of personal problems and an overwhelming feeling that I must get as much as possible into my life in case it was cut short. I was forty one when I discovered complementary therapies and started to search for a natural alternative to warfarin. I had the most success with traditional Chinese herbs. I started training to be a reflexologist, and I acquired some knowledge and understanding to enable me to slowly improve my own health and well-being. Then I heard about Aly Harrold and the amazing things that could be achieved through health kinesiology. I started a course of HK sessions with her.

At this point Aly takes up the story:

Margaret's first issue was entitled *Boosting My Self Esteem And Confidence* and the second was *Harmonising The Subtle Bodies.* Her hot flushes and headaches started to improve and, after about six weeks, the headaches stopped completely and Margaret had more energy, but still there was no change in the prothrombin reading. (Prothrombin is one of the body chemicals involved in blood clotting.) The next issue was *My Role As The Supporting Parent*. The name of the issue was important to Margaret: she had raised her sons Keith and Stewart as a single parent. Five months after her first appointment Margaret's dose of warfarin had been lowered by 1mg per day. We were starting to head in the right direction! Margaret also reported having had no hot flushes at all.

Our fourth issue was *Taking Control And Encouraging Permanent Prospering*. (The title of the issue again was important to Margaret. Her health prevented her getting life insurance regarding a mortgage, and she planned to move house at some point). The fifth issue was called *Generating Healing Energy And Restoring Balance To The Pulmonary Blood Supply*. This was exciting, as it was the first issue which gave a direct reference to our goal. The final issue was *Facing My Fear Of Relying On Others*. Muscle testing indicated it would be five months for the work to have its full effect. This proved to be correct, because five months later Margaret started to have intermittent nose bleeds. (An indication that the blood is too thin caused by too much warfarin). Margaret took only three more doses of warfarin over the next two weeks, and then no more.

The result of a blood test seven weeks later showed that Margaret had no thrombotic tendencies. Margaret is considered now, no more at risk than anybody else of suffering repeated blood clots. Margaret's overall health has generally improved and she has now taken up Morris dancing, something in the past she longed to do but would not have had the energy for!

Client *Margaret Leadbeatter* and Practitioner *Aly Harrold*

Working In Overall Body Sequence

Sometimes the energy system does not want to focus on a particular named area but on several seemingly different areas. This is referred to as working in overall body sequence. In this case, the practitioner does not seek to identify an issue, but works by offering the whole menu of possible techniques and procedures, and allowing the energy system to choose which ones to use. This is like dipping into several different books in the library and reading a small part of each. The health kinesiologist does not know in advance the exact outcome that will be achieved, but trusts the innate wisdom of the body to produce the most beneficial results. The practitioner establishes what to do first, does that, and then asks what to do next, and so on. Sometimes the different procedures relate to various symptoms, sometimes they may be addressing fundamental energy disturbances.

Meridian Analysis

Meridian analysis is another way of structuring the energy work. The previous three ways (client specified issues, HK tested issues and overall body sequence) are the most common ways of working, but sometimes meridian analysis is most appropriate.

If meridian analysis is chosen, it means that the best way to help the person is by looking at the synchronization, energy and information exchange and feedback between the different acupuncture meridians. As well as energy flowing *through* the meridians, it also flows from the meridian to the cells of the body and *between* meridians, connecting everything in a unified whole.

A good example of meridian analysis is the work I did on Mike Collins.

Mike came to see me because he had been diagnosed as having a slightly over-active thyroid gland. He had been given medication by his GP and that was beginning to help, but the GP was still talking about the possible need for surgery. Mike's first appointment was in July and I did not see him again until the December because his job takes him out of the country a lot.

On the first visit his energy system chose meridian analysis: the large intestine meridian was not able to receive energy and feedback properly from the triple warmer meridian. On the second visit his energy system again chose meridian analysis, but this time the focus was that the gall bladder meridian was not able to receive energy and feedback properly from the triple warmer meridian. The triple warmer meridian is concerned, among other things, with the health of the thyroid. It is interesting that in both sessions the energy system said the problem was not with the triple warmer meridian itself, and by implication not with the thyroid gland itself. The over-activity of the thyroid gland was a symptom of problems elsewhere in the energy system. The problem was with the meridians that should have been receiving energy from the triple warmer meridian: large intestine and gall bladder. So the work we did focused in the first session on making the large intestine meridian able to accept the triple warmer meridian energy. In the second session the work focused on the gall bladder meridian. Another way of looking at this is to say that in Mike's case there was nothing wrong with the thyroid energy: it was hampered in its job because other parts of the energy system were not working correctly, causing an over-energy state in the triple warmer meridian. This fits with the thyroid gland being overactive.

Meta Analysis

Meta analysis is another way of organizing the work, although it can seem rather elusive compared with some of the other methods. It is chosen by the energy system when it wants to look at problems within or between subtle bodies.

"My problem is being resolved by a joint approach of conventional and complementary medicine."

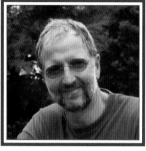

Mike Collins

Over several months I had become aware that I had some form of medical problem but in true male fashion 'thought it would just go away'. Finally my family encouraged me to seek medical advice. Following a discussion with my GP and a blood test, an over active thyroid was diagnosed with the drug carbimazole considered the initial treatment. This was started immediately. Three months later the diagnosis was confirmed by a nuclear medicine scan as 'general over-activity'

Of some concern were the suggested long-term treatments, which were explained as either surgery or radioactive iodine taken as a drink: both would be followed by hormone replacement for the rest of my life. Both courses were irreversible and if I am honest, rather worrying. Following the successful treatment of my wife for a non-related illness I decided to visit Jane Thurnell-Read.

The first session was constructive and interesting, particularly as Jane was able to point to problems away from the thyroid, though associated with it. Having seen my wife treated, I was aware of the nature of the sessions and was not fazed by them and 'went with the flow'. If I am honest, I did not physically feel a difference then or later though the results were positive as blood tests over the period indicated that my medication could be steadily reduced.

The results of the second session five months later were completely different. It is hard to put into words how I felt, however, the session itself was in the same format as the first, lasting fifty minutes to an hour, and at the end I was advised I should feel a lot better in four weeks. The problems indicated by muscle testing were uncannily correct. As I left the building I remarked to my wife that I felt wonderful, euphoric even, but thought that must just be a passing feeling having had a positive consultation. The feeling not only lasted the rest of the day but for weeks afterwards.

My GP reduced my prescription still further, and suggested that we might be able to continue a reduction to nothing, and that surgery and radio-active iodine are very much last resort options. Ten months after my first blood test, a further blood test proved to be normal and my GP reduced my medication to the minimum dose. Seventeen months later I stopped the medication and now haven't needed any for three months.

I would like to think that my problem is being resolved by a joint approach of conventional and complementary medicine.

Client *Mike Collins* and Practitioner *Jane Thurnell-Read*

Human beings are not just physical bodies. Simplifying it somewhat, each one of us also has a series of subtle energy bodies. There is an energy blueprint for the physical body, so that the foetus grows correctly, cells replicate in the correct manner and the physical body repairs itself appropriately. This is known as the etheric body. The emotional body contains our emotional experiences. The mental body is the source of practical day-to-day thought, abstract philosophical thought and imagination. The intuitive body gives us our ability to empathize and connect with others, and the spiritual body contains our sense of the divine.

These different subtle bodies interact and affect each other, and sometimes the most appropriate way to work is by looking at the interaction between these bodies. This can seem a very nebulous way of working, but where it is appropriate, it can produce very definite results, including improvements in physical symptoms. One client came up with *Higher Mental Body Seeing Intuitive Body*. He had problems with one of his ankles. Neither of us understood exactly what this meant, but the work we did based around this certainly did the trick!

Facet Analysis

When the practitioner is working according to an issue title named by the client (client specified issue), or a priority issue chosen by muscle testing (HK tested issue), practitioners will generally then use facet analysis. This ensures that the questioning as to what techniques and procedures to carry out or recommend is as thorough as possible.

Facet analysis is another of the great strengths of health kinesiology. It is a way of making sure that every aspect of a problem is considered, so that the practitioner does not unwittingly impose limits on what is to be done, by having a limited concept and using restricting questioning.

For example:

- It is no use getting rid of someone's asthma if they develop migraines instead, or suppressing an irritating rash so that they develop months or years later a distressing and possibly even life-threatening disease.

- There is some success in stopping a ten-year-old wetting the bed, but it would be even better if the therapist also dealt with the lack of self-confidence and the shame that has built up over the years as a result of this problem.

- It is good if we can stop arthritis getting worse, but it would be even better if the therapist could reverse the damage as well.

- It is better to address the whole problem, so that the symptoms are completely cleared, rather than dealing with only the symptoms.

HK practitioners are trained to be aware of these potential traps and, by using facet analysis, avoid any possibility of falling into them. HK facet analysis makes sure that all aspects of the problem or illness are considered, so that problems are not suppressed or ignored. The HK practitioner looks at the issue from five different viewpoints or facets:

- The cause facet

- The process facet

- The effect facet

- The symptom facet

- The repair facet

In working out what to do the health kinesiologist is not simply looking for the cause of the illness, but also for factors that may contribute in keeping the problem going. For example, an asthmatic may have a cat allergy, although the asthma started before they owned the cat. In this case the cat allergy is not part of the original problem that triggered the asthma, but is part of the process that keeps the problem going, or even makes it worse. Dealing with the original triggers for the asthma without dealing with the cat allergy may, at best, result in only a partial improvement in the client's health.

"The surgeon found no sign of a blockage"

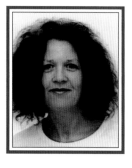

Briony Latham

Jane came to see me because she was suffering from a blocked fallopian tube. She had been for an ultrasound scan, which showed a blockage of one and a half centimetres diameter and she had been told that she would need keyhole surgery to remove it. She was experiencing a lot of pain and discomfort and feeling generally unwell. There were seven energy corrections, an energy toning and an adjunctive to work out. After the work Jane decided to ask for the operation to be deferred for a month to see what would happen as a result of the work. Six weeks after our appointment the operation went ahead, but the surgeon found no sign of a blockage, and Jane has been fine ever since.

Client "*Jane*" and Practitioner *Briony Latham*

Sometimes a client has found benefit from having an illness. This does not mean that they developed the illness in the first place for the benefit, but, having acquired an illness, they found that it had unexpected advantages. For example, the migraine sufferer who found that having a migraine allowed her to be the centre of attention, rather than the 'slave' of her family, needed help to find healthier ways of getting the attention and support she needed.

Health kinesiology protocols, such as facet analysis, allow these factors to be found and handled in a gentle, supportive and professional manner.

Sometimes muscle testing establishes that only some of these facets need attention.

The practitioner first asks:

- Is there any work to be done in the cause facet?

The practitioner asks this question for all the five facets, and then finds what work is needed by offering the menu of techniques and procedures. This is discussed in more detail in chapter 5.

The Cause Facet

In spite of its name the cause facet is not concerned with identifying the cause of any problems, but rather with looking at what work is necessary to counteract the circumstances that triggered the problem initially. The HK practitioner does not necessarily need to know why the problem happened in the first place, but does need to find out what work, if any, is needed to counteract this initial cause.

Health kinesiologists recognize the importance of addressing the origins of a problem, but see it as one part of a much broader perspective. Often the origins of a problem are long gone, but there are processes and effects that keep the problem going, so other facets need to be addressed in order to help a client heal completely.

Unfortunately, western medicine often seems to be over-concerned with identifying the cause of a problem, with labelling and categorizing illnesses and offering standard solutions. Many people have illnesses that have developed an impetus of their own, even though the original cause has long gone.

The Process Facet

Here the therapist is looking at the process that keeps the problem going. The process did not start the problem, but it does keep the problem going. A simple analogy is that of a ball. If the ball is on the flat, it does not move unless someone kicks it, so kicking it is the cause of the ball moving. If the ball encounters a slope after it has been kicked, it will travel further, so the slope can be seen as part of what keeps the ball moving, part of the process.

The climber with the contraceptive pill allergy described on page 35 needed work doing in the process facet for that allergy. The contraceptive pill allergy was not the cause of her bad back – this was due to a fall while climbing – but the allergy was tying up valuable body resources and contributing to keeping the problem going.

Events can occur that reinforce an existing situation. A client lacking in self-confidence, because they were always belittled as a child, may have this lack of self-confidence reinforced by subsequent events, for example a failed marriage or the loss of a job. These events are not the cause of the lack of self-confidence, but may need addressing for the client to feel truly confident.

Many people find an advantage in their illness. They may find that their illness allows then to avoid things they do not like, or to manipulate other people. This does not mean that they deliberately became ill in order to avoid things, but that, having become ill, they have now found their illness useful.

A child with asthma confided in me that he quite liked having asthma, because it meant that he did not have to take part in sport at school. This child had not developed asthma in order to avoid sport, but once he had asthma he had discovered its advantages and was, therefore, subconsciously reluctant to let it go.

If the therapist does not address this aspect of the problem by working in the process facet, then it is possible that the initial symptoms will disappear but will then be replaced by new symptoms. So the child who was using his asthma to avoid sport at school might have developed migraines or recurring stomach upsets, so that he could still avoid sports lessons, if his underlying problem around the sports lessons were not addressed.

A client with migraines said: "In a way I don't want to get rid of my migraines – they tell me I'm working too hard. When I feel one starting I know I need to rest. If I didn't get migraines, I'd probably overwork and die of a heart attack." If I had just worked on the original cause of the migraine, this woman would have surely not got well, when she believed the alternative was a sudden death. Work was needed in the process facet to ensure that she was able to take time for herself and to rest when she needed.

The Effect Facet

Work in the effect facet covers many different situations. For example, if a client has a knee injury, then they will probably start to walk differently. This can cause problems for the other knee, the hips and the back. If HK work is done for the injured knee, so that the client is able to walk properly again, then the problems with the other areas may right themselves spontaneously. If, however, the problem has been going on for a long time, then the other parts of the body may need specific work too. This would be covered in the effect facet.

> I had a client who was very distressed because her partner had started a relationship with another woman. My client was torn between love for her partner and anger at what he was doing. We found an issue title and then used facet analysis. I was surprised to find that her energy system wanted an SET done on her hair (see page 109) in the effect facet. When I remarked on this to her, she told me that her hair had been breaking since the problem in the relationship had started. She was delighted to think that as well as helping her cope with the stress of what was happening, her energy system was also keen to put right the problem with her hair. She was also impressed that I had found this problem, even though she had not mentioned it when I was taking the case history.

The Symptom Facet

Sometimes it is not necessary to do any work in the symptom facet. In some cases, if the practitioner does the work in the other facets, the symptoms will disappear. Yet sometimes, even with all the work in the other facets, work is still necessary here. For example, the symptoms may be extremely stressful for the client, and work needs to be done early on in the treatment programme to give the client relief. Sometimes clients need early evidence of an improvement in their symptoms so that they are convinced of the power of HK.

> One of my long-standing clients gave a friend a one-session treatment from me as a Christmas present. The friend came to see me and it was soon clear that the only reason she had come was because she felt it would have been impolite to refuse her friend's gift. The new client told me of many different symptoms, and I thought that she was likely to need many sessions of work. I also thought that unless I did something dramatic she would not come back again. I asked her energy system if we could focus only on the symptom facet for the first session in order to give her some positive benefit from the one session. We were able to do this. By the end of the session she said "I can breathe through my nose for the first time in thirty years." She was astounded. We had worked only in the symptom facet to give her this immediate and dramatic proof of the power of health kinesiology. Subsequently she herself paid for further sessions with me, and we were able to continue the work started in that session.

The Repair Facet

Work in the repair facet will often speed up the healing process, although sometimes work is needed to ensure that healing does not proceed so fast that it is uncomfortable. This can occur with arthritis. If the body reorganizes the joints too quickly, the person is likely to suffer excruciating pain. This might cause them to abandon the treatment, so wisely the body might add work in the repair facet to slow down this process so that it is comfortable for the client. Sometimes clients do experience pain and discomfort as the healing process takes place, but this does not mean that the practitioner has done anything wrong. It may well mean that this is the only way the body can accomplish the healing.

The organization for a health kinesiology session can seem incredibly complex, but in practice this is not the case. The HK practitioner is trained to be able to complete this analysis quickly and thoroughly, ensuring that the subsequent time is spent in the most effective manner for the client.

"She named the baby after me"

Bridget, aged 44, came to see me for health kinesiology when she was eight weeks pregnant. She had been pregnant seven times, but only managed to have two live births. Her second child was two years old and has Down's syndrome. Bridget's symptoms included a feeling that her head was spinning, an inability to focus properly, low blood pressure, severe exhaustion and nausea. She had had these symptoms in all her previous pregnancies.

Treatment for her included some dietary recommendations: taking ginger root up to week twenty seven of the pregnancy, increasing citrus fruit and foods containing zinc and omitting some foods. I also advised her to take a vitamin C supplement. Everything was tested very carefully for Bridget. Testing also showed that she was allergic to her own progesterone, so we corrected that as well as doing other corrections for her. The result of all this was that within one month the morning sickness improved, and her previously low blood pressure went up to 120/70. She had more energy and was able to drive and go shopping again.

When Bridget was about twelve weeks pregnant, she started experiencing heavy vaginal blood loss from a fibroid on the side of the womb. Treatment this time included various psychological corrections; she also had to increase the dose of some supplements she was taking. The bleeding stopped and the next scan showed no sign of the fibroid.

Bridget had various sessions with me to help her cope with her pregnancy and her concern that she might have another baby with Down's syndrome. Finally Bridget gave birth to a healthy baby daughter. She named the baby after me – Katherine!

Client *"Bridget"* and Practitioner *Cathie Welchman*

5: The HK Menu

Having decided with the aid of muscle testing which of the five approaches to use, the practitioner is then able to offer the HK menu of techniques and procedures, which will allow the focus chosen by the energy system to be addressed. Again the practitioner will use muscle testing to establish which techniques are needed and in which order to carry them out.

The possibilities are divided into five distinct categories or factors:

- Energy correction factors

- Energy redirection factors

- Energy toning factors

- Adjunctive factors

- Environmental factors

Energy Correction Factors

Much of the actual work done by the health kinesiologist falls into this category. Health kinesiology is concerned with rebalancing the energy system at the deepest level, and this is one of the fastest and most effective ways to do this, so it is by far the most important factor. Energy corrections are so powerful that they normally only need to be done once to achieve permanent removal of a particular stress, imbalance or blockage. During a series of health kinesiology sessions a succession of energy corrections allow more and more stresses to be removed from the energy system, allowing the body the energy and space to heal itself.

There is such a range of possibilities for energy corrections that they are sub-divided into categories. Some of the most common ones are:

- Energy control system (see chapter 6)

- Psychological (see chapter 7)

- Allergy, tolerance and symbiotic energy transformation (see chapters 8 and 9)

- Tissue energy blocks (see chapter 9)

- Energy flow balancing (see chapter 10)

The practitioner narrows down the possibilities, by asking first about these categories, and then sub-dividing even further. This sounds like a very complicated process, but HK practitioners are able to do this systematically and quickly.

If the practitioner is working within an issue and has established, for example, that the client needs work in the cause facet for that particular issue, the practitioner would ask:

- Are there any energy control system corrections to do under the cause facet?

If the practitioner is working in overall body sequence, then the question would be:

- Do I do energy control system corrections next?

If the practitioner is using meridian or meta analysis, the question would be:

- Are there any energy control system corrections to do?

If the answer to the question is 'yes', the practitioner then asks about all the sub-categories within the energy control system correction factor. If the answer is 'no', the practitioner asks about other categories, such as psychological, SET and energy flow balancing. When the answer is 'yes', the practitioner again asks about the sub-categories within that factor.

Often the client will need several different types of corrections, so a typical course of treatment could involve doing some energy control system corrections, some psychological corrections and some work on detoxifying the body and correcting allergies. In addition, work in the other factors - energy redirection, energy toning, adjunctive and environmental - may also be needed.

The Basic Format For Energy Corrections

All energy corrections involve the same basic procedure:

- The practitioner identifies the stressor through muscle testing

and then

- The stress is triggered in a controlled manner

and at the same time

- The practitioner removes the stress permanently by rebalancing the energy system via the acupuncture meridians.

This combination of triggering a stress and rebalancing the energy system is referred to as an energy correction, or just a correction.

The exact way in which this is done varies enormously. For example, triggering the stress can involve the client thinking something, touching themself, or having magnets, homeopathic remedies or crystals placed on their body. The possibilities are endless and sometimes involve two or more of these possibilities at the same time.

Sometimes the tasks necessary to trigger the stress do not make sense at first, and even seem bizarre and unreasonable. One such correction happened during a workshop. To trigger the stress one student had to smell the breath of another. When we came to do the correction, both participants burst out laughing. Using muscle testing I established that the correction actually was for spontaneous laughter. In its wisdom the energy system knew that 'laugh spontaneously' is an impossible instruction for most people, so the correction got set up in a bizarre way so that spontaneous laughter was the inevitable result.

Holding Acupucture Points And Using Cosmic Batteries

Once the stress is triggered the practitioner rebalances the energy system through the acupuncture meridian system. This is achieved either by lightly holding a combination of acupuncture reflex points or by using one or more of the devices known as cosmic batteries, while the stress is in place. This enables the energy system to overcome the stress and eliminate the disturbance it was causing.

Holding acupuncture points does not involve needles, or even the practitioner applying any pressure. Sometimes the practitioner will ask the client to help hold points, as this allows the procedure to be completed more quickly. Most

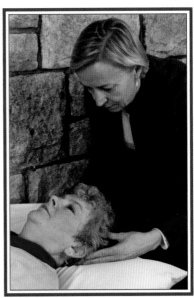

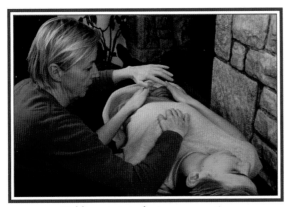

Holding points during a correction

More points that might be held during a correction

acupuncture points can be held through clothing, so most clients find it a really gentle process.

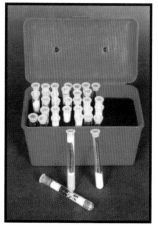

Cosmic batteries

Often, instead of holding acupuncture points the practitioner will test to see if cosmic batteries can be used to rebalance the system. There are thirty-four of these glass tubes each containing, among other things, symbols, metal coils and homeopathic tablets. When used correctly, they have the property of doing the same job as holding points, that is, to rebalance the energy system. Clients will frequently report that the cosmic battery feels cold or warm or heavy, even though it will be at room temperature and is, in fact, very light.

It is very convenient if these can be used, because in general they allow the work to proceed at a faster pace than when acupuncture points are held. Sometimes they allow the practitioner to undertake corrections that would be difficult to carry out if acupuncture points were being held. For example, on occasions energy corrections can involve the client moving in some way, and then it can be very difficult to hold precise acupuncture points at the same time. In these and similar circumstances cosmic batteries are an extremely useful piece of equipment.

As always, muscle testing is used to establish exactly which points on the body to hold or which cosmic batteries to use and where they should be placed. The cosmic battery or batteries are often simply placed on the torso. If the client needs to move or is a wriggling child the batteries will be temporarily taped in place while the correction is completed.

Touch Localising

Before beginning the correction process the practitioner will usually want to double-check that the right stress has been found. This is done using a process called touch localising, often abbreviated to TL'ing. The stress is triggered, and then the muscle is tested while one or more specific points on the body are touched. If the trigger does indeed stress the person, the arm muscle will test weak. This is a way of confirming the verbal questioning.

This test is carried out again at the completion of the correction to check that the arm muscle now tests strong, and that the item is complete. The practitioner will then double-check that everything is correct by asking the question:

- Is this item completely and robustly done?

Once the energy correction is completed the practitioner will then go on to the next item or group of items.

Energy Redirection Factors

Although the bulk of the work carried out by the practitioner is under energy correction factors, the client may also need work under the energy redirection factor.

In energy redirection items the client may need to touch a specific part of their body, or think a specific thought, while acupuncture points are held or cosmic batteries are placed on the body. They look very similar to energy corrections, but their effect on the energy system is different. Here the practitioner is not removing a stress, but directing energy to some specific purpose.

Energy redirection techniques are used when the energy of the body needs to be directed to some specific goal that may not be of the highest priority for the body. Of course, this is only undertaken after the body has given specific permission to do so.

> Some HK students had given me a pair of earrings, and, as I put them in, I caught my ear on one of the wire hooks. The ear started to swell and become hot and red. I quickly tested what needed doing and performed an energy redirection procedure and the ear returned to normal - much to everyone's relief. It was a simple technique carried out in a matter of minutes: I had to hold the damaged part of the ear between two fingers while a cosmic battery was placed on my torso. This focused the attention of the energy system on the problem allowing rapid healing to take place. In terms of my overall health it was a very trivial problem, but I asked my body to heal it, because the students were distressed that a present they had bought for me was causing me discomfort.

On several occasions I have used this technique to help to remove skin tags. While not a real threat to health, these can be unsightly and annoying.

> In a class demonstration for focused energy redirection Sheila Bracewell volunteered. She had a skin tag on the right side of her neck. This was a nuisance as it caught on her collar and jewellery. For the energy redirection she had to place her fingers on the tag while two of the class members held the relevant acupuncture points. After a short time the tag beneath her finger started to hurt with a sort of prickling sensation. A day later the tag was already smaller and in three days it had disappeared completely.

Energy redirection procedures are also used when the body seems to be stuck in a rut. Changes have been made, either through HK energy corrections, or through outside circumstances changing, but the body is still running in the same old groove. The new healthier options are available, but for some reason the system seems unable to recognize them.

I used an energy redirection procedure to good effect on a Dutch lady, living in Germany. She was extremely fluent in Dutch, German and English. Unfortunately she spoke so quickly that people had difficulty understanding her, regardless of what language she was using. One of her German friends told me: "It's like being shot with a gun when she speaks!" We used an energy redirection technique on her and within a couple of hours her speech rate had slowed right down, much to everyone's amazement and amusement. She told me that both her mother and her older sister spoke very quickly, so possibly when she was small it had been important for her to speak quickly in order to have a chance of speaking at all! The energy redirection technique reminded her that circumstances had changed, and the behaviour that was advantageous as a small child was now causing her problems in her relationships as an adult.

Energy correction factors and energy redirection factors are procedures that are carried out during the session, but three other categories - energy toning factors, adjunctive factors and environmental factors - usually involve the client doing things after the session.

Energy Toning Factors

Energy toning factors are activities that the person goes away and does to tone their energy system. Aerobic exercise tones the physical body, energy toning tones the subtle bodies (see page 49). As with physical exercise, energy toning exercises are usually done repeatedly to strengthen the energy of these bodies. Common energy toning activities include:

- Affirmations, where the client has regularly to repeat a positive statement (see page 139)

- Visualizations, where the client visualizes something; for example, a colour or themselves achieving what they want (see page 140)

- Taking flower remedies, such as the Bach Flower remedies (see page 138)

- Carrying crystals (see page 139)

- Performing energy toning exercises (see page 141)

Adjunctive Factors

Adjunctive factors are also activities that clients do for themselves. Whereas energy toning affects the physical body through an **indirect** route, adjunctive factors affect the physical body directly. Adjunctive factors include:

- Nutritional supplements (see page 135)

- Physical exercise (see page 137)

- Rest (see page 136)

- Wearing magnets (see page 137)

Environmental Factors

Environmental factors cover reactions to environmental problems. This includes problems of environmental pollution and toxicity and also geopathic stress problems. Geopathic stress occurs where the earth's energy field is disturbed. This can result in ill health for people who live or work in such areas. My book *Geopathic Stress: How Earth Energies Affect Our Lives* looks at this problem in detail.

The five factors - energy correction, energy redirection, energy toning, adjunctive and environmental factors - cover a rich and varied range of techniques and procedures. It is not possible within the confines of this book to cover all the different possibilities, but the following chapters give an insight into these powerful tools, which can help so many people to be healthier and happier than they ever dreamt was possible.

6: The Energy Control System

All energy corrections have the same basic structure of triggering an energy disturbance, while rebalancing the energy system. Each aspect of the energy system is prone to particular types of disturbances, which need to be specifically triggered. To put it another way, different ways of triggering the disturbance will work on different parts of the system. Energy corrections can, therefore, be divided into different categories according to the way in which they affect the energy system, and the part of the energy system they work on. One of these parts is the energy control system.

The energy control system (ECS) can be described as the mail delivery system of the body, but instead of delivering letters it delivers information and energy. The energy it delivers is not physical-type energy, but what in Chinese medicine is called life-force energy or Chi. Corrections involving the ECS are often the first thing that is needed: the delivery system has to be functioning correctly. Other types of work, such as psychological corrections or SET, ensure that the messages being delivered are correct.

Energy control system corrections are a sub-category of one of the five main factors – energy correction factors. The energy control system can be faulty in various ways, so there are different types of correction procedures for different faults. Some of these corrections are covered in this chapter, and some more in other chapters: mechanism control corrections (chapter 9) and scar corrections (chapter 11).

The ECS corrections can affect the physical body in many different ways, e.g. speed up healing, reduce pain and inflammation. They can also help people emotionally and lead to improvements in clarity of thinking, concentration and memory. At first it may seem strange that one category of corrections can have so many different effects, but this is because ECS corrections are correcting problems in the fundamental messaging function of the energy system.

Electric Current Corrections

Electric current corrections are needed when there is metal in the body, and a weak electric current has been set up that interferes with the body's own electrical signals.

An electric current is generated easily when there are two dissimilar metals in an electrolyte. Such a situation can arise in the mouth. The saliva is the electrolyte – a very good conductor of electricity – and dental amalgams are composed of several dissimilar metals. Measurement of these minute electric currents in patients with at least two or three amalgam fillings has shown that the electrical output involved is a thousand times greater than that used by the body in nerve conduction (Robert Hempleman *International Journal of Alternative and Complementary Medicine, November 1997*). Although the electric current generated would be of no interest to the National Grid, it does appear that in some people it is enough to interfere with the brain's activity. This can lead to headaches, behavioural problems, an inability to concentrate, think clearly and remember things.

A similar problem can also occur with dental braces, which are made of several dissimilar metals. It is sad that many teenagers wear dental braces during the critical years before their GCSE exams. Dental braces could lead to these children not succeeding as well as they should, because the electric current generated by the brace may interfere in the activity of the brain.

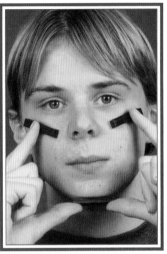

Fortunately, using the rather fearful-sounding electric current correction, the health kinesiologist can usually solve the problem caused by amalgam and dental braces. The correction is very simple. It involves placing several magnets around the mouth and rebalancing the system by holding acupuncture points, or placing cosmic batteries on the client's body. The electric current correction does not seem to stop the battery-effect being there, but it does stop the client being excessively disturbed by it.

Magnets in place for an electric current correction

I had treated two children in a family with great success, so, when one of the children suddenly became dyslexic overnight, the mother decided to consult me. When the child came in to my office, I noticed that she had a brace. I asked her mother how long it had been since the dentist had fitted the brace. Her mother told me it was six weeks. I then asked when her daughter had suddenly become dyslexic. This was also six weeks previously. Through muscle testing I established that my surmise was right – she needed a simple electric current correction. This took a maximum of ten minutes. That evening her mother telephoned me - she was very excited. She told me that she had gone to pick her daughter up from school as usual, and the child's teacher had made a point of speaking to her. He told the mother that it was as though a switch had been thrown, because the child's sudden dyslexia had completely disappeared. He asked her what had happened in the morning, when the mother had taken her daughter out of school – he was in no doubt that this was the cause of the child's dramatic transformation.

As well as creating problems, amalgams and dental braces can also make existing symptoms worse.

A boy of twelve was brought to see me. He had been suffering from migraines for some years. He was wearing a full brace. When I questioned his mother she said that his migraines had started before the brace was put in, but that they had become worse since he began wearing it. The solution to his problems was not just a single electric current correction, as happened with the previous child, but an electric current correction was part of the work needed to clear his migraines.

I have also noticed that nearly all the clients who have come for help to stop biting their nails need an electric current correction as part of the treatment. I am not sure why this is the case, but it certainly often forms part of the usually successful programme of work for these people.

The modern fashion for body piercing can have serious side effects. Body piercing only seems to be a problem from the point of view of electric currents when there are body fluids involved. Body fluids are excellent electrical conductors, whereas normal skin is not. Tongue and genital piercing, for example, may cause problems, but eyebrow piercing will usually not cause a problem that needs an electric current correction. Piercing in any area of the body can, however, cause other problems, which are corrected usually by scar corrections (see page 130).

The epileptic teenager described on page 106 came back to see me again. She told me that she had experienced seven to ten fits in the previous week after being fit-free for over two years, following her previous HK treatment. I established through muscle testing that having her tongue pierced two weeks before was largely to blame. Fortunately for her we were able to use the electric current correction so that she could keep her tongue stud and become fit-free again.

Sometimes electric current corrections are needed when the client has metal in other areas of the body. One client had shrapnel in his arm from the Second World War, and that required an electric current correction. Another client had metal in her replacement hip joint and this was causing problems. In these cases the magnets are placed in close proximity to the metal in the body.

Some people can undoubtedly have metal in their bodies without any problems, but for the vast majority it seems to be a problem. It is usually a simple matter to put the problem right.

Electromagnetic Field Corrections

Electromagnetic Field (EMF) corrections are needed where the body's own electromagnetic field is disturbed in some way. It is not always clear why this happens, but trauma and accidents of even a minor nature can certainly cause disturbances that need this type of correction. The correction process is very similar to that for electric current corrections, but this time the magnet or magnets can be placed anywhere on the body, as identified by testing, while the system is rebalanced.

HK practitioner Franky Kossy helped a client who had developed eczema, while watching his older sister dying of cancer. He had never had any skin related problems before, so the family all assumed the eczema was a response to the stress of the situation. Franky offered to see if she could help. Muscle testing revealed that EMF corrections were needed, with magnets around the affected area. By the next day the eczema had already started to retreat and within a few days it had completely gone. Using EMF corrections for eczema is not common, but through muscle testing Franky was able to establish that this was exactly what was needed.

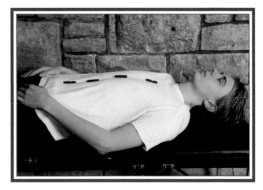

Getting ready for an electromagnetic field correction

Spin Corrections

Energy in the meridians flows in a particular direction. For example, energy in the stomach meridian flows from the second toe to a point just below the eye, and in the bladder meridian begins by the bridge of the nose and ends by the nail of the smallest toe. As well as having a direction of flow, energy also spins, rather as a bullet spins as it travels through the air.

The meridian energy in healthy living tissue should spin in an anti-clockwise direction, but if the energy spin is disturbed, one or more spin corrections may be necessary.

The spin correction can be done in several ways. One possibility is for the practitioner or the client to make small clockwise or anti-clockwise movements with a finger over the specific spot or spots on the body where the energy spin disturbance is occurring. Another possibility is to use life transformers (see page 139) – usually either the ones for protection from geopathic stress, or the ones for protection from electromagnetic pollution.

HK practitioner Shahzadi Thomas saw a client who was complaining of severe shoulder pain. Spin corrections came up. Shahzadi worked out the exact locations for the two items, and stood behind the client's shoulder spinning her fingers. Suddenly the client said: "Oh my goodness! Something very strange has just happened. It was as if the pain just slithered away down my back, and now my shoulder feels fine."

Phantom Sensation Corrections

Phantom sensations seem to occur because the energy blueprint of a part of the body remains, even after the part has been removed. Sometimes the person may feel pain, tingling or numbness, and a sense that the tissue is still there, even though it is not. Phantom sensation corrections look very similar to scar corrections (see page 130), but are done for a different reason. Normally the client places a finger or fingers over the area where the body part is missing. The exact location is established by muscle testing, and the practitioner holds acupuncture points or places cosmic batteries on the client to complete the correction.

> A client phoned me and asked if I could help her. She had been to the dentist two weeks previously for an extraction and was now in excruciating pain, in spite of taking antibiotics for a week before and after the extraction. She was having to resort to painkillers and was extremely distressed. I arranged an emergency appointment for her and quickly established that the pain was because the energy system had not recognized that the tooth had been removed, so she was still suffering from the toothache associated with the tooth. I did a simple phantom sensation correction and one electromagnetic field correction with a magnet placed on her cheek. When I next saw her, she told me that the pain had gone very quickly after the session.

Alignment Corrections

Alignment corrections are necessary when the body processes are not co-ordinated at an energy level. Each part may be working perfectly, but the co-ordination is not good, so the whole process does not work. This is equivalent to mail being sent by the central sorting office to the local office **after** the postman has left to deliver his letters, so the mail has to wait another day.

An alignment correction can be quite complicated to set up - there are four components to the correction:

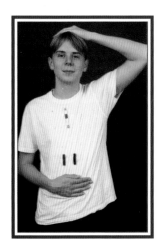

Standing ready to have an alignment correction carried out - the person will also be thinking something specific

- The client has to think something.

- The client has to touch their own body, usually with both hands.

- One or more magnets are placed on the body.

- The client has either to be in a particular position (e.g. standing, sitting or lying), or to do something specific (e.g. holding the breath in or closing the eyes).

The precise nature of each component is established using muscle testing. Only when all the components are in place can the correction begin. As usual the practitioner holds acupuncture points or places cosmic batteries on the client's body.

Jayne Bartlett worked with a client for several months. In one of the later sessions Jayne completed an energy alignment correction and muscle tested to establish the benefits that the client would experience. She found that the client was expected to notice improvements in her digestion, sleep and the condition of her hair. She would also feel calmer and more focused. When Jayne next saw her, the client reported that she had experienced all of these improvements. She was particularly pleased, because her manager had encouraged her to apply for promotion. The client felt that the confidence in her expressed by her manager was as a direct result of the work Jayne had done.

BBEI Corrections

A particularly powerful yet simple technique in health kinesiology is the BBEI correction. BBEI stands for body brain energy integration, and this wording reflects the fact that this type of disturbance affects the connection from the body to the brain.

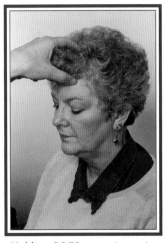

BBEI corrections deal with primitive fears, set up in early life, that hinder the smooth transmission of energy between the body and the brain. These primitive pre-language fears begin either in the womb or during birth or before two months of age. I suspect that after two months of age the baby's brain is sufficiently developed to stop the possibility of distressing events affecting its functioning in this way. Although these are fears, they do not include phobia-type fears such as a fear of spiders. Phobias are psychological fears and are corrected using psychological procedures (see page 83).

The BBEI correction procedure is very simple and straightforward. The practitioner has a list of the most common BBEI items. Having established, through muscle testing, which of the items need correcting

Holding BBEI correction points

during the session, the practitioner holds the specific BBEI reflex points while the client thinks the words, for example *fear of not being free*. The client thinks these words over and over again; sometimes the words will generate images or emotions, sometimes they will not.

Examples of typical BBEI items:

– *fear of being abandoned*
– *fear of not being loved*
– *fear of not being able to know what I want*
– *fear of not being able to breathe*
– *fear that I won't be good enough*

Obviously the foetus or baby does not think in these terms: this is adult wording for these primitive feelings. When the client thinks *fear of being abandoned*, for example, it recreates energy stresses similar to that experienced by the baby or foetus.

BBEI fears can be set up as the foetus or young baby responds to its environment. People usually have many of these types of fears. This does not necessarily mean that they had a difficult start in life, but simply reflects the baby's inability to analyze and understand what is happening. For example, when the baby is hungry, it does not have the concept that this will only last for a short time because someone will feed it, so *fear of hunger* can be set up. If the bedclothes accidentally cover the baby's face, it does not have the ability to remove them, and so *fear of suffocating* can begin.

BBEI fears can also start because of the mother's experiences. The psychological stress of the mother gets transferred to the foetus and a BBEI fear starts for the baby.

> Practitioner John Payne saw a ten-year-old boy, who had difficulty going to bed and sleeping. Various corrections were done including a BBEI *fear of being falsely blamed*. At first his mother said: "Oh yes, that seems just like him; he's always saying he gets blamed when it's his brother's fault." After a few moments she said: "It could be more about me, because, when I was pregnant, my husband and his family blamed me for almost everything. I couldn't do anything right almost from the time we met." The child soon stopped being difficult about going to bed.

> Julie Flower went to see practitioner Sandie Lovell. As part of the work Sandie found that she needed to do some BBEIs on Julie. One of these was *fear of water*. As Julie started to think the item, she started to see detailed images of three children in 1940's style clothes, playing in a pond with a tractor tyre as a makeshift boat; the little girl fell into the pond and was very upset, as she could not swim. Julie subsequently found out that her mother had had such an experience when she was six years old, but had never told anyone about it.

BBEI disturbances can have a profound effect on behaviour, and that effect will be felt virtually from the beginning of life, because of the age at which they are set up. The effect of removing them can also be profound.

This is particularly true if an individual has several opposing items. One client had a long list of BBEIs that needed correcting, including *fear of life* and *fear of death*. She also had *fear of bright lights* and *fear of darkness*. Not surprisingly, she was a depressed person. I explained that part of the reason for her depression was probably because she had these opposing fears, which left her with no viable options as to how to arrange her life.

Sometimes BBEIs make perfect sense in relation to the client's problems or behaviour. Many asthmatics need a correction for *fear of suffocating* and *fear of not being able to breathe*. Overweight people often have *fear of hunger*. People who feel the cold and take lots of clothes with them even on short journeys in the middle of the summer often benefit from a correction for *fear of being too cold*. People who have difficulty forming lasting relationships need the BBEIs *fear of needing others* and *fear of being hurt emotionally* corrected.

I had one client who talked non-stop. I (and I suspect everyone else) found this very exhausting. Correcting BBEIs involve the person thinking of the fear. Each time I asked this client to think an item she would do this for a few seconds and then start talking about it. I had to keep reminding her to **think** the item rather than talking about it. Eventually through muscle testing we came to a new item: *fear of silence*. We corrected this item – in silence – and then we completed all the succeeding ones – in silence. This is a clear example of the power of the BBEIs. This client had a fear of silence from very early on in her life: one way of avoiding this fearful situation is by talking all the time to fill the silence.

BBEI corrections are taught right at the beginning of HK training. On the second day of her training one student had the BBEI *fear of rejection* corrected. At lunchtime a group of us were going out to lunch together and she was included, but she went to the toilet first and we inadvertently went without her. When we came back to start the afternoon class, she told us that she had been amazed at her reaction to this event. Normally she would have felt that we had deliberately gone without her, because we did not like her. This time she realised that it had happened totally unintentionally, and so she was disappointed but not desperately hurt and upset. She also told us that she had been adopted as a small baby and had felt rejected by others all her life. She said that normally she would have been so upset she would have gone into a shell and withdrawn into the background, still with the feeling that she was not liked. Now she felt this pattern of behaviour had been broken and she had great hope for the future.

BBEI corrections can dramatically improve relationships. Imagine the situation if you have *fear of bright lights* and your partner has *fear of darkness*; you have *fear of being too cold* and he or she has *fear of being too hot*; you have *fear of noise* and he/she has *fear of silence*. How would you agree on how to light and heat your home together? Your partner would come in from work, walk into the sitting room, switch the CD player on, then perhaps immediately go into the kitchen and switch on the radio, then upstairs to the bedroom to get changed accompanied by the sound of the bedroom TV. The lights would be left on in every single room and all the windows would be opened to cool the house down. You would come in shortly afterwards and switch off the CD player, before going into the kitchen and doing the same thing to the radio. You might then go into the bedroom to be greeted by the remark: "I was listening to the CD – why did you switch it off?". Many serious relationship problems can begin at this simple level of incompatibility. Dealing with the BBEIs – a simple HK procedure – allows these problems to be eased.

One client reported an unexpected improvement after we had corrected *fear of being shaken*. Her boyfriend was a very fast driver and would be constantly braking and swerving to overtake other cars. This always led to arguments on a long journey.

After having this particular BBEI corrected, she found that she could go on long journeys with him without problems. I suggested to her that she should try to get him to come in for an appointment to help him be a safer and less aggressive driver.

"No further problems with her feet"

Louise had frequently suffered from aching feet on standing or walking during the past three to four years – the right was worse than the left, and they were worse in warm weather. Her job involves her in a lot of standing so it was a real problem for her.

In the session I only did three BBEIs:

– *fear that I can't love others*
– *fear of being noticed*
– *fear of being cared for*

Two years later she told that she'd had no further problems with her feet since that first appointment.

Client "*Louise*" and Practitioner *Sue Davies*

BBEI fears look very similar to psychological problems, but because they are set up very early on and affect the energy feedback from the body to the brain, they are tested for and corrected in a slightly different manner from psychological corrections. Yet they are not completely separate. In fact practitioners repeatedly see situations where a BBEI fear is set up early in life and subsequently reinforced at the psychological level. In order to help the client, the practitioner has to unravel this combination of BBEI and psychological effects. It may well be that because a fear already exists at a BBEI level, relatively minor emotional events carry more weight and then get set up at a psychological level. When the practitioner finds a BBEI item for a client, the client will often identify an event that they think triggered it. The event is often in childhood or early teens – much too late to be a BBEI – but the event may well be so memorable because of the pre-existing BBEI stress involved.

The HK energy control system menu includes a variety of different correction procedures – the ones discussed in this chapter are some of the most commonly used ones. These procedures may seem totally unrelated to each other, but what they have in common is that they are all concerned with the messaging system of the body. It is no good only ensuring the messages are correct; they need to be correctly delivered too.

Ensuring correct delivery is the job of the energy control system corrections. They often lay the foundations for the rest of the work, or sometimes these corrections can give dramatic results in their own right.

> Practitioner Frank Kossy saw a young man with hearing problems. He was mentally handicapped and lived in a residential home. He had been given a hearing test, which indicated impaired hearing, and there were plans to fit him with hearing aids in both ears. His mother knew he would not wear hearing aids, so she took him to see Franky. Using the mother as the surrogate for muscle testing, they performed the necessary energy alignment correction. As the young man left the room, his mother called after him and he turned around. The residential home has not re-tested his hearing, but they do not feel he now needs hearing aids.

"He looked at me like I was mad."

It was the night before my check-up for my hearing – my hearing test – and I just felt my ear pop – not a pop but like a pop. It felt more like something opened in my ear and then I could hear clearer.

The following day when I went for my hearing test they told me there was nothing wrong with my ears. I told him about the HK because he wanted to know how come it's better now. When I told him I was having health kinesiology, he looked at me like I was mad, but said to carry on with whatever I was doing.

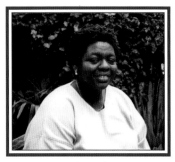

Jennifer Robinson

Everything just sounds clearer and I can tell which direction traffic is coming from. On the telephone with my right ear it used to sound like they were far away, so I always used my left ear. Now I can use my right ear and it sounds like they're shouting!

I used to fall over in the street suddenly, for no reason. I would fall over in the street and my daughter would say: "Mummy, get up." Since my hearing got better that hasn't happened once. I don't know if it's because my ears are better, but I think it must be.

Client *Jennifer Robinson* and Practitioner *Sally Smith*

7: Psychological Corrections

One of the great strengths of health kinesiology is its armoury of psychological corrections. An HK practitioner's work with a client will often involve a series of different types of psychological corrections. Often physical problems will respond to psychological work. There are two reasons for this: many physical problems have a psychological component, and psychological stress can take up so much of the body's energy that there are not the resources left to deal with the physical problems.

Rob Adams, a practitioner in Chester, saw Mrs Prince, a teacher in her fifties. She had developed a shoulder problem. Rob is trained in remedial massage and manipulation as well as health kinesiology. This seemed an obvious case for remedial massage and he expected to be able to put it right in two or three sessions, but did not succeed. Mrs Prince's doctor offered her a course of physiotherapy, with no more success. She then came back to Rob again, and this time he used HK. On looking at the corrections that came up it was evident that she was worried about her imminent retirement and did not know how to cope with it. Treating her psychological stress proved to be the way forward rather than dealing with the physical problem directly. She has now been free of all symptoms for two years.

Sometimes clients are initially worried at the idea of dealing with psychological matters, but they quickly realise that health kinesiology offers an extremely safe environment in which to deal with even deep psychological traumas. This can be done quickly without having to discuss painful and deeply buried experiences. The health kinesiologist does not have to delve into the client's past. The client does not need to reveal all or apportion blame.

Long-standing stresses and traumas can be dealt with, empowering the client to make new decisions. Health kinesiology work does not **make** the client do anything, but by removing the stress from certain thoughts and situations it allows the client to think more clearly and make appropriate decisions for themselves. Health kinesiology does not change reality, but it can and often does change how people deal with reality.

A good example of this occurred during a workshop. One of the students was explaining the problems she and her family were having over the location of a fish tank. As she described the problem, it became very clear that the fish tank needed to be put in another room. This was such an obvious solution that I assumed that there must be some good reason why this could not be done, so I did not mention it. The HK work was carried out to remove the stress. When she came for the next workshop, she announced triumphantly that she had solved the problem of the fish tank by moving it into another room. The other students were, like me, taken aback that she had not thought of this simple solution before. She and her husband had been so stressed by their disagreement over the fish tank that they had been unable to see the simple solution that suited everyone. Once the HK work had been done, the student was no longer angry and upset; she could think about the problem in a rational manner and see the obvious solution.

I don't know how it's gone but it's just gone.

The main reason I went to see Jane was because I had a horrendous problem with jealousy, which made me very obsessive and too difficult to live with. I had experienced a very painful marriage that ended in divorce. I had spent fifteen years on my own because I was so afraid. Then my current partner, Keith, came into my life. I fell in love with him and the whole thing started all over again. He is a therapist and spends much of his life with women. This pushed every button in my body, though he had done absolutely nothing to deserve this. I became obsessively jealous and thought I was going mad. Then Jane appeared and did the trick.

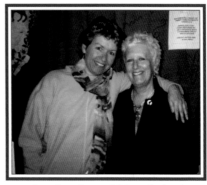

Jane Lumley and Mary Richard

I worked through it fairly fast and by the end it had just gone. I don't know how it's gone but it's just gone. We worked on fears and trust and so many different things. I saw her for - I don't remember how many sessions - each time something different would come up. I think over a period of about three months I went from horrendous jealousy to total peace in that area. The thing that amazed me was how painless it was. I had to do odd little bits of homework - usually an affirmation or doing some small exercise – it would last for perhaps three days. I didn't have to keep working and working and working - the incredible ease of the process, I found that so remarkable.

Client *Mary Richard* and Practitioner *Jane Lumley*

The Basic Format Of Psychological corrections

There are almost thirty recognized types of psychological corrections, so this book can only explain some of these, but almost all follow the same basic format as other corrections: a stress is identified through muscle testing, and triggered, while acupuncture points are held or cosmic batteries are put on the body. In the case of psychological corrections, the client must **think** about something, or repeat a word, phrase or sentence to themselves to produce the stress. The practitioner uses muscle testing to establish exactly what the client needs to think. This thought can spontaneously generate pictures, emotions, intellectual connections and sensations in the body. Sometimes the client cries or laughs.

Clients can usually readily accept that a negative expression, such as *experiencing sadness*, can be stressful, but people are often surprised when muscle testing shows that *experiencing happiness* or *love* or *contentment* is also stressful. However, the reasons for this are quite straightforward. Many people feel they do not deserve happiness, because they are not good enough, or because there is so much suffering in the world. They may feel that they do not deserve love, or that it is a big responsibility to be loved by someone. Contentment may seem boring, or undeserved, or unbelievable.

While a person has negative or ambiguous feelings about a positive state, they will be stressed by thinking about it and will not seek to achieve that state wholeheartedly. Removing the stress does not instantly make the person happy, contented or full of love, but it allows them, if they wish, to pursue these goals vigorously, and perhaps to be less disturbed if they are unobtainable.

Clients are sometimes surprised when items such as *not being loved* come up. They may say that they do not **want** to be happy about not being loved. I explain that sometimes they are going to be in situations where they are not loved - for example when a close relationship ends, or when they reprimand their children. The HK work will help them cope with these types of situations.

Sometimes clients worry that this will lead them to be selfish and unkind to others. In fact, the reverse is usually the case. Once these stresses are removed it is easier to see what is needed and find non-manipulative ways of achieving it. Clients often find they can also experience more genuine concern and understanding for other people.

Another worry that clients sometimes express is that the psychological corrections will make them behave in a certain way rather than being themselves, but HK psychological corrects liberate people to be more truly themselves by giving them more non-stressful choices about how to conduct their lives. Psychological corrections do not turn introverts into extroverts, for example, but they do seem to smooth the rough edges off our personalities.

Psychological corrections can also be used very successfully for animals. In this case the owner or the practitioner thinks the thought while they touch the animal.

Practitioner Sandra Herrmann worked on her rabbit, Benny, who sometimes had fits of anger and aggression. Sandra's flatmate was frightened of Benny, and he even attacked some builders as they walked through the garden. Sandra decided to see if HK would help. She told me: "Normally when he senses that I am up to something, he runs away, but this time he stayed, obviously waiting for something. I worked out only one psychological correction: *I am important.* I thought the words for him, and when the correction was done Benny ran off again. The same evening, my flatmate commented on the change of behaviour in Benny. Since then he has not tried to bite anyone and is now just as affectionate as any other rabbit."

Finding The Exact Thought For Each Item

The thought could take one of many forms. They may need to think about something or someone, or to repeat a specific key word or words to themselves. I have had a client who had to think about tapioca pudding – evocative of school dinners and childhood unhappiness – and clients who have had to think about dying. The possibilities are endless. It is often impossible to find the items intellectually, although they often make perfect sense once they have been found. So the HK practitioner needs a systematic way of narrowing down the possibilities.

Many psychological corrections that involve the client thinking a word or phrase are categorized according to their grammatical structure. This categorization is not arbitrary: it is clear that different types of grammatical structures work in different ways. These different types include:

- Being/not being corrections (see page 77)

- Gerund corrections (see page 78)

- NV (I) item corrections (see page 79)

- Imperative corrections (see page 80)

- Linked opposite corrections (see page 81)

- Phobia corrections (see page 83)

The practitioner begins by establishing which grammatical structure is to be used. Next, the exact number of items has to be found, and the precise wording for each item established. For some structures there is a list of possibilities that have been previously used, and the practitioner simply tests to identify the ones needed by asking questions, such as:

- Is the first item in the first column of the list?

- Is it between here and here? (Pointing to the places on the list.)

The client is not necessarily aware of what is on the list, but the muscle testing will still allow the correct items to be identified.

For structures with no list of established items the practitioner has a more complex task to find the exact wording. Sometimes intuition on the part of the practitioner or client will suggest all or part of an item, but these intuitions are always then tested for their accuracy. At other times practitioners ask systematic questions to establish the wording, such as:

- How many words are there in the item – at least three?

- Are any of the words an emotion?

- Is the second word 'my'?

The practitioner may use a dictionary or a thesaurus to help track down the precise word. Practitioners may also use other types of word lists, such as lists of verbs or abstract concepts, to help this process. So, for example, the practitioner can ask:

- Is the first word on my list of abstract concepts?

- Is the third word on my list of prepositions?

These are different lists from the ones mentioned earlier, where the whole item is on a list – these word lists contain single words rather than complete items.

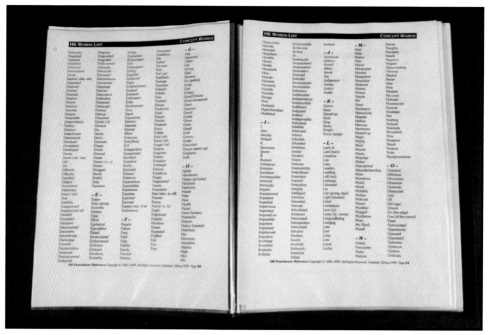

A working manual open at a words list page

Sometimes the issue title and/or the client's symptoms can give clues to what the words might be. A client who suffered from persistent bloating came up with an issue title: *Happiness*. The psycho-logical items were:

– *I bloat when I'm unhappy*
– *I dream of being happy*

A client whose husband had died produced these three obviously relevant items:

– *Frozen desolation*
– *Unbearable desolation*
– *Never-ending desolation*

There are many different psychological corrections. The ones discussed here have been chosen because either they come up frequently or to give an insight into the range and richness of psychological corrections.

Being/Not Being Corrections

The being/not being correction is one of the most powerful within health kinesiology. The client first has to think *being A* and then *not being A*. *A* can be a single word or a phrase. Clients who need this correction are often stuck in some area of their life: whatever behaviour they adopt in that area is stressful. For example, someone who is stressed by *being happy* and also stressed by *not being happy*, will neither be totally at peace, when they are happy, nor when they are not happy.

Someone who is stressed by the idea of being loved and also stressed by the idea of not being loved, is likely to have difficult relationships where love is involved. They may relate well to their boss, their acquaintances, people in shops, their accountant, and so on, but any relationship were there is the dimension of love, such as sexual relationships and family relationships, is likely to be fraught. When they feel loved, they are stressed by that and so start to move away from that situation, but then they move into not being loved and are stressed by that, so they move back towards the being loved arena, and so on. This constant yo-yoing is exasperating for anyone trying to love them: one moment they appear to be seeking love and the next minute rejecting it. They may even end relationships to avoid the stress of being loved, but then the stress of not being loved becomes ascendant. Again they start their search for a loving relationship, only to rebuff it when they find it. Being/not being corrections can resolve this internal conflict and the resulting inconsistent behaviour. By removing the stress both from *being loved* and *not being loved*, the practitioner gives the client more non-stressful options to choose, and also the ability better to cope with life when it is not as they wish.

People who need a lot of being/not being corrections are often depressed. This is not surprising, because they find that they are in a no-win situation. Whatever they do takes them towards one of the situations that stress them, even if it takes them away from another stressful situation. Being/not being corrections can remove them from this no-win situation and allow them to behave in a more rational manner. Then they are likely to achieve more positive outcomes in their life.

Gerund Corrections

The gerund corrections are some of the most commonly occurring psychological items in HK. A verb ending in '–ing' is known grammatically as a gerund, and is the first word of each correction. Sometimes the same gerund is common to all items in a group:

- *Accepting peace*
- *Accepting love*
- *Accepting forgiveness*
- *Accepting happiness*

Sometimes the gerunds are different and the words that follow are common:

- *Trusting myself*
- *Liking myself*
- *Believing in myself*

As with all psychological corrections, the client has to think each of the items in turn while the system is rebalanced.

Sometimes the items that come up are apparently obscure, but sometimes they relate directly to the problem the person has. A small child was brought to see me because he was not sleeping very well and spent most of the night in his parents' bed. The items, clearly reflecting his worries, were:

- *Fearing fear*
- *Fearing darkness*
- *Fearing silence*
- *Fearing emptiness*
- *Fearing loss*
- *Fearing rejection*
- *Fearing separation*
- *Fearing danger*

Once these and some other items have been corrected, he began to sleep well in his own bed.

One young client had moved house and, because the new garden was much smaller than before, his pet dog had gone to live with his grandparents. He was extremely unhappy, and his parents were most concerned about him. Some of the items that came up were:

- *Missing my friends*
- *Missing my dog*
- *Missing my house*
- *Missing my garden*

A long-standing female client came to see me. She had started a new relationship and was extremely excited by this, but also anxious as to whether it would last. Some of her items were:

- *Being aflame*
- *Being wanted*
- *Being golden*
- *Being spoilt*

Sometimes the items are almost poetic in the way they are constructed:

- *Leaving my fears appeased*
- *Leaving my worries soothed*
- *Leaving my apathy behind*
- *Leaving my childhood resolved*

As with all psychological corrections, the client has to think each of the items in turn while the energy system is rebalanced.

Christine Emery saw a woman who had been suffering from palpitations on and off for two years. The client told Christine that the problem had started after she had experienced a bad reaction to some ecstasy. All but one of her friends had left her when she was having the reaction, and she had felt very sick and frightened. Christine did three psychological items: *feeling abused, feeling very abandoned* and *feeling apathetic,* and also got her to think about the events of that evening while she held acupuncture points. The client rang Christine eleven days later to say that she was about seventy five per cent better, and that this was the first time anything had helped the problem.

NV (I) Item Corrections

The NV of the name stands for neuro-vascular points. These are a particular type of reflex points that are always used for this type of correction. The (I) part of the name is because these items usually start with the pronoun 'I'. These corrections help to prevent the destructive and paralysing dialogue with ourselves that we all engage in from time to time:

I will do it.
I won't do it.
I can do it.
I can't do it.
I must do it.

This sort of seesaw thinking keeps us stuck and stressed and unable to move forward. A typical group of items could be:

- *I am happy*
- *I'm not happy*
- *I should be happy*
- *I won't be happy*
- *I can't be happy*

The procedure for correcting these items has an additional step to the standard process. As usual the item is corrected by the client thinking the item while the acupuncture energy system is rebalanced. Once this has taken place, the client is instructed to make 'a tent' with their fingers. A drop of a solution of choline, a B vitamin, is placed in the mouth and, with eyes open, the client thinks: *It is OK that I* ..., completing the sentence with the previous words, for example, *It is OK that I am happy.* HK practitioners do not know why this additional step is necessary for this particular type of correction, but it does seem to make it a more robust correction.

> Celeste Jones used the NV (I) Item correction to good effect when working on a teenage girl who was very depressed and had refused to attend school for the last week. She reluctantly agreed to see Celeste. Celeste found various corrections including: *I need help*; *I should have help*; *I am helped*; *I must have help* and *I ought to have help*. The next day she was a lot brighter and went back to school again. Over the next few weeks she became increasingly positive and started to talk about how she was feeling, instead of keeping everything inside.

Imperative Corrections

These psychological corrections have two different possible qualities. There are items that sound like imperatives or commands, and others that sound more like pleas. Examples of the first type are:

- *Be good!*
- *Grow up!*
- *Behave!*
- *Be careful!*

These seem like echoes from childhood, the sort of things said by adults to disobedient or thoughtless children. When they come up for adults, it suggests that the words and feelings of these reprimands are still affecting the client, even as an adult. Sometimes the problem is that the client is still obeying these commands. Sometimes the client is rebelling against them. In either case a client affected in this way is not truly in charge of their own life.

Sometimes it seems that the messages come from childhood, not as actual verbal commands, but rather as unspoken messages understood from adult attitudes and beliefs about how to behave. For example:

- *Be unhappy*
- *Reward negativity*
- *Don't do what you want*

Clients will often recognize that even though their parents or other influential adults never articulated such things, the way they lived their lives and interacted with others gave these sorts of messages.
Examples of imperative items that sound like pleas are:

- *Understand me*
- *Love me*
- *Protect me*

In this type of imperative item it seems to be the client who is pleading for understanding, love, or protection.

Regardless of what quality the imperative items have, they are corrected in the same way as other psychological corrections.

Linked Opposite Corrections

Linked opposite corrections seem to help us deal with apparently primal conflicts. They are constructed of two words joined by 'and'. The first word is positive, and the second word opposes it in some way. Examples of these include:

- *Abundant and irresponsible*
- *Alive and numb*
- *Coherent and destructive*
- *Creativity and work*
- *Deserving and poor*
- *Loved and divided*
- *Organized and dry*
- *Power and worry*
- *Worthy and degraded*

"Miraculously the acne had just about cleared"

When I first started my practice at a new clinic, another therapist referred a client with acne to me because she was having no success. Nicole had suffered from acne from age eleven, and, although living in France, still came to England regularly. Both cheeks were covered with acne that had been there for at least twenty years with no sign of ever leaving. I worked out a client specified issue, which included BBEIs and a few psychological corrections, including some linked opposites. We blitzed through a two-hour session as she was leaving the next day to return to France.

On her way to the ferry Nicole stopped in at the clinic to show me that miraculously the acne had already begun to clear. Over the next few months and several visits for other issues her skin continued to get better and even the scarring started to disappear.

Client *Nicole Ryan* and Practitioner *Franky Kossy*

I originated this correction myself and am very proud of it. It came about because I was concerned at the lack of progress in some areas of my own life. HK had helped me in so many ways – long-standing and seemingly intractable symptoms had gone – but there were still some major aspects of myself that I wanted to improve. I became convinced that a new correction would enable me to address these problems – and the result was the linked opposites correction. Originally I thought the list of possible items would be endless, and I recorded the examples I found with clients in order to give other practitioners some ideas of the type of items that were likely. However, it became apparent very quickly that there are only a limited number of these items, possibly because they represent archetypal conflicts and tensions. So there is now a standard list of linked opposite items, which practitioners use to establish the correct items for clients.

When the linked opposite list was translated into German for the students and practitioners who work in that language, it became clear almost immediately that only certain words worked; a direct, literal translation often did not work, so the translation had to be carefully checked through muscle testing to make sure each item had the right energy quality.

This energy quality is perhaps best described as a tension. It has been likened to that experienced when two magnets are held together with the same poles facing: repulsion and a sense of the sameness of the energy is experienced simultaneously.

It is not always clear why the energy system chooses a particular item, but sometimes the obvious rightness of the items can be startling. For example, one client had been talking to me about her feelings about being adopted. When we started working, her energy system produced the item *chosen and different*. Another client needed the item *alive and empty*. She had miscarried several times and was now trying to become pregnant again.

Phobia Corrections

A phobia is an extreme, irrational fear – in fact it is so irrational that even the person suffering from it will usually recognize that the level of fear is unreasonable. Phobias can have a big influence on people's lives, causing them distress and limiting what they are able to do.

Edith Watson had a phobia of bridges, flying and heights. She travelled on planes but was not happy. Her husband had retired, and they were planning the holiday of a lifetime to New Zealand. Practitioner Josie Donaldson saw her twice for this. Edith sent postcards to Josie from around the world saying the phobia had almost gone. She had eleven long flights, one helicopter flight and a two-hour flight in a very small plane. Two of the flights involved mishaps and emergency landings, one of which was a wheel bursting on take-off. She had no problem with bridges over very high gorges. She was thrilled, and her husband was amazed and impressed with the change in her attitude to travel.

HK has specific phobia techniques, but they are not necessarily the way to address a phobia. The lady with severe agoraphobia discussed on page 113 did not need these specific techniques to help her overcome her phobia.

The HK phobia correction consists of a group of items. Each item is very carefully selected through muscle testing. The first item is the least demanding. Once that is corrected the next item is found and corrected. This procedure is repeated until the client no longer has the phobia. Each item needs to be stressful enough for the client to benefit from the correcting process, but not so stressful that the client will refuse to do it. The procedure involves the client thinking or doing something related to the phobia while acupuncture points are held or cosmic batteries are placed on the body.

An example might be:

– *Imagining a cat in the next room*
– *Imagining a cat in this room*
– *A real cat in the room being held by someone*
– *Imagining touching a cat*
– *Touching a real cat held by someone else*
– *Touching a real cat that is not retrained in anyway*

Because the items are carefully chosen through muscle testing, this technique is very safe: the client is taken through the stages at a pace that they can cope with. The results of this procedure are often quite remarkable.

Some years ago I had a client who wanted to fly to her son's wedding in Barbados. She had always suffered from claustrophobia and was terrified of the thought of the flight. She had two appointments for health kinesiology treatment. After the first appointment she found she could think about the trip without getting in a panic. After the second appointment she flew to Barbados and sent a postcard to me: "Had a good flight, no problems - I wasn't the least bit nervous. I got fed up after five hours but no claustrophobia."

"She was totally happy and excited"

Barbara came to me for sessions, because she wanted to be able to drive, but she had a deep seated fear of being in a car. As a child Barbara had repeatedly had the same nightmare about sitting in a car. This car was driving without her; she had no control over it, and this driverless car at the end of the dream had an accident. Then she always woke up totally wet from sweating and frightened.

When she was eighteen she obtained her driving licence with a lot of stress. She was able to pass because the driving instructor sat next to her in the car, so she did not have the full responsibility to drive, because if something happened, he still could interfere and help.

Barbara was able to drive – but it was always a major drama – and even then, only, if someone was sitting next to her. Because of the dramas involved it was no pleasure for her to drive, so she gave up driving.

When she was thirty three she wanted a new job, but for this job she needed to be able to drive a car, so she needed to face her biggest fear and get rid of it.

In the first session I tested out and corrected quite a few general fears. In the second session we did phobia corrections:

– *seeing herself in a car, when someone else is driving and she sits in the back of the car*
– *seeing herself in a car, when someone else is driving and she is sitting next to him*
– *seeing herself driving a car, when someone else is sitting next to her*
– *seeing herself driving a car, when someone else sits behind her in the car*
– *seeing herself driving a car alone etc.*

Barbara sweated a lot, and she felt she could not move her right leg and foot to use the gas-pedal.

The third session involved various corrections including some EFB corrections (see chapter 10), where she sat on a chair and simulated driving, and I had to make movements and/or noises from various angles to correct her abilities to respond to the movements and/or noises whilst driving.

Afterwards we had to drive in my car, with Barbara holding certain reflex points, whilst I was driving. She had to watch me: what and how I did while driving. Afterwards she drove in the little streets through the vineyards next to my practice.

As homework Barbara had to drive, with someone with her in the car, finding times in the day, when there was not so much traffic. I tested exactly, how she should 'build up' her driving, e.g. driving the first time alone early on a Sunday morning, when there are not much cars around etc.

For her fourth. session Barbara drove herself alone in her own car. She was totally happy and excited, and although she was still trembling, she did it. We made a few other psychological corrections around trusting, relaxing, letting go. Afterwards she drove home happy and relaxed, looking forward to starting her new job, having finally solved a main problem theme in her life.

During the second session Barbara told me that she was born in a car, as her parents could not make it to the hospital in time. Her mother nearly freaked out giving birth in the car: situations like this are only funny in a Hollywood movie but not in real life.

Client "*Barbara*" And Practitioner *Eva-Maria Willner* (Germany)

A Psychological Session

Usually a session or issue will contain different categories of corrections, but sometimes a session is devoted entirely to psychological corrections.

A client in her twenties had decided to live with her boyfriend. She was extremely apprehensive about this, and her existing health problems were becoming worse because of the stress. The move would also involve leaving her pet cat with her friends, and she was feeling very sad about this. Her energy system chose an issue title *Safety or Marriage*, and we did a series of psychological corrections:

    – *Living is difficult*
    – *I have to start living*

    – *Resisting freedom*
    – *Resisting change*
    – *Resisting uncertainty*

    – *Abandoning my cat*
    – *My cat dying while I am living elsewhere*

On her next visit to me five weeks later she told me all her physical symptoms had improved and she was feeling very well and happy. The HK work had helped her to come to terms with her anxieties.

"She said 'I'm hungry.' She has an excellent vocabulary but this is a word she had never used."

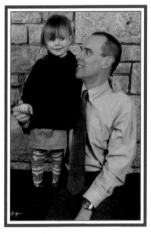

Emily Manley and John Payne

It was recommended that I take Emily to see John by someone he had treated - she thought he was marvellous. Because Emily's problem was about constipation I didn't want to go down the conventional medical line, because I didn't want anyone messing with her. I felt she was too young to understand what was happening, but old enough to know it was something she was not enjoying. So I made an appointment with John.

Three appointments later we had solved two problems and I was absolutely amazed and started recommending John to everyone I thought had a problem in life. Really it was an ongoing problem: she'd never ever been much of an eater; she didn't feed well as a baby; she wasn't good on solid food. She was absolutely tiny like a little doll. She had been constipated since she had been on solid food – sometimes it was so painful it made her scream. She would feel nauseous when the constipation was bad. There was no pattern to it. It recurred frequently and she could take days to settle down afterwards.

When we left after the first appointment she said "I'm hungry." She has an excellent vocabulary but this is a word she had never used. I took her to McDonalds and she ate everything – we've never looked back. The first night after the appointment she had horrific nightmares, so I phoned John who was very reassuring. Within a couple of days the constipation was as bad as ever – Emily was screaming again. I phoned John and he said to bring Emily in to see him. Now it was time to deal with the constipation. Various things came up that she must have got from me while she was in the womb. Again she was quite still while the corrections were done.

Now (five months later) she will eat something at every meal and has a different attitude to food. She has no constipation, although sometimes it's harder than others. She's a different person with food and I'd say there's been a 30% increase in her body weight since she first saw John. She's so much less stressed – it had begun to take over her whole life. I can now start nappy training her.

Client *Emily Manley* (this piece is written by Emily's mother, Sarah Manley) and Practitioner *John Payne*

Psychological corrections form a large part of a health kinesiologist's day, whether they are just part of the work done, or make up the entire programme of work. Long-standing emotional stress can be resolved quickly and safely, and work in this area leads to improvements in physical well-being, energy levels and often seemingly unrelated symptoms.

8: Allergy And Tolerance

Jimmy Scott, the founder of health kinesiology, defines allergy as:

"any energy disturbance in response to exposure to a substance. The substance could be a food, cosmetic, chemical, animal hair, pollen, mold, etc. ... With allergy the energy system reacts to **any** amount of the substance."

This is not the same as the medical definition of allergy, which emphasises the involvement of the immune system rather than the energy system: "a collection of conditions caused by inappropriate or exaggerated reaction of the immune system to a variety of substances." *The British Medical Association Complete Family Health Encyclopedia*.

The terms allergy and intolerance are sometimes used interchangeably, but in health kinesiology they are not the same and each term has a precise meaning.

Jimmy Scott defines tolerance as:

"the amount of the substance the body can handle without becoming stressed" and "There is a tolerance limit for everything, no matter how wholesome."

Allergies Are On the Increase

More and more people are suffering from allergic reactions to a huge range of substances. Inhalers for asthmatic children are now commonplace in primary schools. Steroid creams for eczema are available over the counter. Processed foods often give warnings that they may contain traces of nuts for people with nut allergies.

Many people decide to try health kinesiology in the first place because they have heard that it can not only detect allergies with ease, but also correct them, so that the offending substance is no longer a problem. Often, even though friends or family have told them this, they are deeply incredulous that it is possible to switch off an allergic reaction permanently. Yet there are many satisfied health kinesiology clients who know that to be the case.

What Can People Be Allergic To?

It is possible to be allergic to anything and everything. Contrary to popular belief it is not just wheat, dairy products and 'junk foods' that cause problems. Some people believe that it is not possible to react to organic products, but others with hay fever, asthma and allergic rhinitis are reacting to organic grasses and moulds. There is nothing that is safe for everyone. For example, I have treated:

- A child who became hyperactive on eating carrots, including organic ones.

- An asthmatic who was allergic to non-biological washing powder but fine on the biological ones.

- A migraine sufferer who reacted to decaffeinated coffee but not to regular coffee.

- A child with eczema who was allergic to cotton, but fine with synthetic materials.

While these sorts of cases are definitely the exception, they do illustrate the point that nothing can be categorized as non-allergenic.

"He can buy his wife flowers"

Geoff Dillow is a poultry farmer in his sixties. He has suffered with allergies to feathers, household dust, pollen and certain chemicals found in some food and drinks.

He has immobile cilia syndrome, which is a lung problem (his lungs being unable to clear the dust and pollen he breathed in). This caused him to suffer with bronchitis in the winter. To help him with this problem his wife would help him drain his lungs at least once a week. On specialist doctors' advice antibiotics

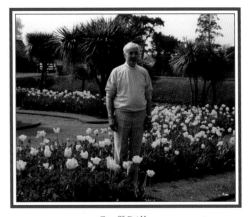

Geoff Dillow

had to be taken three days a month. These upset his stomach, which was as bad as the bronchitis.

After having eight sessions covering a wide range of corrections his wife has never known him so fit. He can now work in the poultry houses, taking just the normal precautions. He can also buy his wife flowers, which he could not do before, because of the effect of pollen in the house. His immobile syndrome is so much improved that he now takes no medication

Client *Geoff Dillow* and Practitioner *Rob Adams*

The Difficulty of Detecting Allergies Without Muscle Testing

If the onset of the allergic response is rapid, detecting the allergen is usually not a problem. The well-publicised cases of anaphylactic shock are an extreme example of this. This is a life-threatening allergic reaction. Massive amounts of histamine and other body chemicals are released, causing immediate changes to the tissues: the blood vessels dilate, causing a sudden lowering of blood pressure, and the swelling of the tongue and airways can precipitate choking and suffocation. When this happens, it is usually easy to identify the problem substance – peanuts, shellfish and bee stings are common culprits.

Sometimes a pattern in the occurrences can suggest the culprit. A child who was persistently wetting the bed, but only in summer, proved to be allergic to pollens. Once that was corrected her bed-wetting stopped.

Often, however, the reaction is not immediate, or the person is exposed to the substance continually, so that the reaction is always there. When the person is allergic to several different substances, or one substance occurs in several different guises, detecting allergies can be difficult without techniques such as muscle testing.

> I once tested a small child who had eczema and established that he was allergic to oranges. His mother replied that she knew this was not true as she had tried removing oranges and orange juice from his diet, and his symptoms had not improved. I carried on testing other things and found he was also allergic to milk. Again his mother said this could not be right, as she had excluded milk from his diet without any success. I then asked her what he had drunk when she excluded orange juice from his diet, and she replied that he had drunk more milk. She also realised that when she had excluded milk from his diet, she had given him more orange juice. She then recognized that my testing could be correct.

A health kinesiology practitioner will not only test for food allergens, but will also look at things the client is inhaling, touching and using at home and in their work. Personal care products, household cleaning materials, fabrics, washing powders, pollens, moulds, house dust mites are just some of the things that commonly cause problems.

Some chemicals are widely used in different industrial processes. For example, the chemical benzene is found in tobacco smoke, petrol, synthetic fibres, plastics and rubbers, inks, oils and detergents. Most HK practitioners have a range of test kits in order that they have a wide variety of substances to test, including these sorts of chemicals. Sometimes it is necessary for the client to bring in specific substances, for example, the hair of the family cat, a favourite perfume or deodorant, and so on.

Sometimes people are allergic to things they encounter regularly at work. I have treated a bank clerk who was allergic to the dye in some bank notes, a priest who was allergic to wine including communion wine, and hairdressers allergic to chemicals in the products they use in their work.

Brian Thornton, a dentist from Southsea, consulted Susan Spencer, a health kinesiology practitioner in Bognor Regis, because he was allergic to the latex gloves he needed to wear in his work, and they gave him a spotty rash. She used techniques specifically designed to counteract the allergy and also other techniques to strengthen his liver and reduce stress. Brian is delighted with the improvement in his hands. He has also found that the hay fever, which he has suffered from since he was eighteen, improved after just one session devoted to it.

Sometimes different substances will produce similar symptoms at different times, and this can make the detection process more complicated.

One client had severe sinusitis all year round. Muscle testing showed that the smoke from her coal fire was affecting her in the winter. It also showed that she was being affected by moulds for most of the year, and that she was reacting to pollen in the summer. She had told me that she could not be allergic to pollen as she had her symptoms all year round, but testing showed otherwise.

Sometimes clients do not even realise that allergies are responsible for their symptoms. A number of clients with appointments in the summer have come in blowing their noses and apologizing that they have 'a cold'. When I ask them how long they have been suffering, they often say for several weeks. I point out that a cold would not last that long and suggest we do some testing. These people are almost always allergic to pollens. They are surprised, because they think that pollen allergy results in itching eyes and sneezing as well as a running nose. Once the pollen allergy is corrected their 'summer cold' quickly disappears – some clients even find that their runny nose stops before they leave my office.

One client tested as reacting to anaesthetics and subsequently told me that she had found it difficult to recover from even minor surgery. On the most recent occasion the nurses had removed the mattress from her bed to stop her lying down during the day. They felt that she was being a hysterical hypochondriac when she insisted she was not well enough to get up after a minor operation. When I explained that she was allergic to anaesthetics and suffering a debilitating reaction, she was relieved to know that her experiences were 'real' and not a hysterical response as people had assumed.

There have been times when the outcome has surprised me at least as much as the client.

A lady with trigeminal neuralgia telephoned me to make an appointment for allergy testing. Trigeminal neuralgia is an extremely painful condition involving one of the facial nerves. It causes a severe, stabbing pain in the face. At that time I specialized exclusively in detecting and correcting allergies. I had no experience of trigeminal neuralgia, and, as none of the literature suggested it could be connected with allergy problems, I dissuaded the caller from making an appointment. A week later she telephoned again and said that she really wanted to be allergy tested, even though she knew I did not think I would be able to help her. I agreed to see her, and testing showed she was allergic to lead. She designed and made pewter boxes, so was exposed to lead in her work. Once we had corrected this her trigeminal neuralgia disappeared completely. I was both surprised and delighted. This client taught me a valuable early lesson about the perils of prejudging situations and illnesses.

Although allergies are being increasingly recognized, there are still many cases were allergies do not seem a likely cause of the problem, until muscle testing reveals the link.

Klaus Schäfer, a teacher and practitioner in Germany, saw a nineteen-year-old client with bulimia. She also suffered from panic attacks at night. She had been bulimic since she was twelve years old and had already been treated in several hospitals. Klaus found that she was allergic to all dairy products and asked her to stop eating them at least for the time being. Three days later she called to say that she was eating normally and had not suffered any further panic attacks. A week later she returned for another appointment and told Klaus that all her problems had returned. It took a little while to find out what the problem was, but he eventually discovered what had happened. The client had gone to see a nutritionist who had told her that as she was not eating dairy products she must stop being a vegetarian and start eating meat in order to get enough protein. Klaus found that she was allergic to all animal protein. He had not checked this during the first session because he knew she was a vegetarian. Klaus then tested a complete diet programme for her and once again her eating problems and panic attacks vanished.

Sometimes a client does not **want** to recognize that they have a particular allergy problem in spite of all the evidence.

A client insisted he was allergic to peanuts, which muscle testing did not confirm. He continued to insist that he was allergic to peanuts and that my testing had been faulty. I re-tested the peanuts on several occasions throughout the session, but each time I got the same answer: this man was not allergic to peanuts. I tested a range of other substances and found that he was actually allergic to hops, which were in the beer that he drank at the same time as he ate peanuts. He was horrified when I told him that he was allergic to beer and not peanuts, and immeasurably relieved when I told him that we could correct the problem for him!

When there are no obvious patterns, and the situation is complicated by many different factors, it is fortunate that muscle testing offers a simple, non-invasive, direct method of testing for allergy problems.

Allergy And Tolerance

To complicate things even further, sometimes reactions are not actually allergies, but are evidence of low tolerance instead. In this case it is the **quantity** eaten, or contacted, that is important – the person only has a reaction when they **exceed** their tolerance level.

It is probable that we all have tolerance levels for everything, but if the tolerance level is for twenty oranges a day then in practical terms this will not matter. However, if the tolerance level is for one small orange, whenever a large orange is eaten problems will be experienced. This situation can be mystifying without this understanding. Clients will remark, for example, that sometimes they can eat an orange and they are fine. Another day, if they eat an orange, they will experience problems. This situation could indicate a tolerance problem. Another possible explanation is a problem with a pesticide or something else connected with oranges. Sometimes tolerance levels are so low that in practical terms the effect is no different from that of an allergy. However, it is different in terms of what is happening in the energy system, and so has to be tested for and corrected differently.

Detecting Allergy Problems

Jimmy Scott developed a sensitive, reliable method of testing for allergy problems. First of all the person is balanced in the normal way. Next the substance is placed on a specific point about two finger widths below the navel. A specific acupuncture point just in front of one of the client's ears is touched, while a muscle is tested. If the muscle tests weak, this means that the person is allergic to the substance placed on their body. In this way a whole range of substances can be quickly tested.

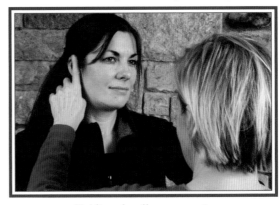

Holding the allergy test point

One of the great strengths of this test is that the client does not have to eat, inhale or be in contact with a suspected allergen – the substance can be in a glass container or wrapped in paper, if convenient. This is extremely important if the person is suspected of being severely allergic to the substance under test. The test works because it is the way the energy properties of the substance interact with the person's energy system that is being tested, not the physical properties of the substance. Often the practitioner muscle tests the answer to some verbal questions first to narrow down the range of substances to test or even identify the actual substance. The test with the substance

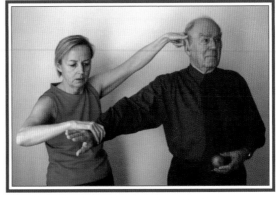

Allergy testing a client – this can be done standing, sitting or lying down

on the body is then used as a confirmatory test. This allows the practitioner to home in on obscure offending substances much more quickly.

These simple procedures allow a whole range of substances to be tested quickly, painlessly and safely.

Detecting Tolerance Problems

When people have tolerance problems, the quantity they consume is important – they only have a problem when they exceed their tolerance, whatever that happens to be. Because this is a different process to allergy, there is a different way of testing for it, although there are also certain similarities.

Once again the client is balanced, and the substance is placed just below the navel, but this time the **quantity** used is important. A specific place on the back of the client's head is touched at the same time as the muscle is tested. If the muscle tests weak, this indicates that the quantity of the substance being tested exceeds the current tolerance level. Quantities can be decreased to determine exactly at what point the tolerance level is exceeded.

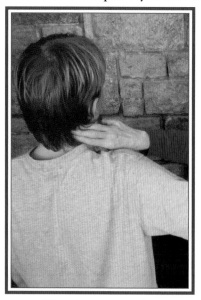

The tolerance test point

This is a very clear test of tolerance levels, but it can also be very messy. A giggle from someone being tested for their milk tolerance level can result in milk being slopped all over them. Also it only tells the clients what their **current** tolerance level is, and that will depend on how much of the test substance they have already eaten or been in contact with recently. In addition, some things, such as exposure to pollens, house dust mite or environmental chemicals, cannot be meaningfully measured in this way.

Because of these considerations the practitioner will often establish tolerance levels by using verbal questions such as:

- Does this person usually have a tolerance problem with milk?

- How much milk on average is it safe for them to drink each day – at least half a pint?

- If the person also has cheese, does this reduce the amount of milk their body can tolerate?

By a process of detailed questions and muscle testing, the exact level of tolerance can be pinpointed.

Many clients are totally amazed about this simple method of detecting allergies and tolerance problems. They become even more excited when they realise that HK also has simple procedures for correcting allergies and increasing tolerance levels.

"It really does work!"

Chloe was born by emergency caesarean section; she never settled after her birth, rarely slept and cried constantly. After many GP visits a specialist diagnosed dairy product allergies and she was put on a special pre-digested non-dairy milk formula. Chloe coped with this until her first birthday.

Chloe, at twelve months, resumed her high-pitched, non-stop crying pattern – and was awake during the whole of every night. As she was on the special milk formula the GP said there was nothing more to be done – but to "put up with it"! By this time Chloe had stopped eating solids, had diarrhoea and did not sleep; she screamed for long periods of time and we were exhausted.

Eventually I took her to see Sandra Shackleton. Sandra identified various allergies and intolerances for Chloe on the first meeting. Sandra asserted that the special milk formula was absolutely no good for Chloe and advised us to put her on to sheep's milk and boiled water. Sandra sorted out various issues for Chloe, psychological and pre-birth – all to be treated during various stages to come.

The first evening of the new diet she slept from midnight to 5 a.m. – and this improved until she now sleeps from 8 p.m. to 6.30 a.m.! Chloe has put on weight and is a happy little girl. Chloe still attends Sandra occasionally to resolve any new issues – but we have no doubt that without our attending Sandra, our baby would now be very ill.

My husband is not particularly interested in complementary therapies; he is a practical man and was sceptical. However, he insisted on meeting Sandra personally, to thank her overwhelmingly for helping the baby to recovery – and restoring harmony in our home – enabling us to have our lives back. He still has no idea how it works – but he stipulates – it really does work! We would recommend this non-invasive, yet powerful treatment to anybody – from babies to old age pensioners.

Client "*Chloe*" (this piece is written by her mother) and Practitioner *Sandra Shackleton*

Correcting Allergies Using The Tapping Technique

In health kinesiology there are two direct procedures for correcting allergies: allergy tapping and the symbiotic energy transformation (SET) procedure.

The tapping technique is an extremely safe and easy technique to learn. Firstly the practitioner begins by checking for energy permission to correct the allergy. Sometimes permission is not given the first time, because other work needs to be done first. Sometimes the tapping technique will not be effective, and the practitioner is only able to correct the problem using the SET technique.

As the name implies, the technique involves tapping various acupuncture points while the substance is placed on a specific point on the body. Usually only one substance can be corrected at a time, but each substance normally takes less than twenty minutes to correct.

A sixty five year old lady, who had been deaf in her right ear for many years and had recently become deaf in her left, phoned practitioner Amina Vierk. Amina found the initial phone call and taking the case history during the first appointment extremely difficult, because she had to shout so much. Testing showed that the client was allergic to dairy products, and that was corrected on her first visit. When Amina saw her two weeks later, the client said that on the sixth day after the appointment she had felt something move in her head when she stood up after bending down. At the time she was looking after her grandchildren and, even before she was standing totally upright, she realised that she could hear her grandchildren talking to each other in normal voices. She had sat in a chair and listened for five minutes without saying a word, because she could not believe that she could hear so well.

If the client has many different allergies, or the energy system does not immediately give permission to correct them, the practitioner may teach the client an adaptation of the technique that can be used when an allergic reaction is experienced. This does not correct the allergy, but it minimizes the discomfort that it causes.

Health kinesiology practitioners can simply but spectacularly correct allergies so that the client no longer needs to worry about the problem.

A woman consulted Pat Ward for a severe allergic reaction to eggs. Even the small amount of egg in, for example, mayonnaise would cause severe stomach pains. After treatment she wrote to Pat: "Thank you for revolutionising my food consumption after suffering more than twenty years!". Her stepson also saw Pat and found that his headaches where attributable to food colourants and antibiotics in milk. Since his treatment he has had no further problems.

Pat also helped a client who was on a very restricted diet because of her allergies: "Eight years living on oats, Ryvita, salad and vegetables". A leading allergy consultant had told her that she would have to learn to live with her allergies. After seeing Pat she found all her allergies disappeared and she could eat a wide range of foods again.

"I am now, at the age of 72, fitter than I have ever been in my life."

I have had bronchiectasis (a serious lung condition) since I was a small child, and an increasingly spastic colon for a number of years. I consulted Jane about seventeen years ago, because I had always suffered from what I recognised as allergies, and these were becoming so severe that I was afraid that I would become unconscious one day, possibly when I was driving my car, or on the stairs.

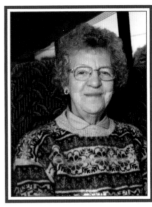

Margaret Bunt

As a result of Jane's treatment, both my long-term problems have greatly improved, the spastic colon having almost vanished, and it is clear that a lot of my symptoms were related to my tendency to produce allergies or intolerances. Perhaps because of my chronic and incurable chest condition, it has proved difficult to balance my system completely, and I still have allergic/intolerant reactions from time to time, though much less often and much less severely than I used to. On many of these occasions, I can myself stop the reaction and desensitize my body to the offending substance, by using the technique of tapping some of the surface-points of the acupuncture meridians in the way that Jane has taught me. For instance, I stopped a very severe reaction to an antibiotic several years ago, and recently reversed an intolerance to some tablets which I had been given to reduce my blood pressure. (I now have some treatment from Jane that we hope will so reduce my B.P. that I shall not need to take medication for it.) I am now, at the age of 72, fitter than I have ever been in my life.

Client *Margaret Bunt* and Practitioner *Jane Thurnell-Read*

Switching off a reaction is extremely helpful if someone is allergic or intolerant to a food, but even more important if the problem is caused by something that it is impossible to avoid: house dust mite or pollens or many industrial chemicals, for example.

One of my clients had been coping with severe respiratory problems for over twenty-five years when she consulted me. She had had conventional allergy testing at the hospital, which had pinpointed problems with house dust, hay, barley dust, cats and dogs. She knew about some of these problems already, but did not want to get rid of her animals. She used a mask and sunglasses in order to cut the grass. As well as having breathing problems, her nose was blocked and her eyes itched constantly. She was using three different types of medication, but still had symptoms all the time. By her sixth appointment she was able to report that her ventolin pump had lasted for two months rather than the normal two weeks. She was using the other medication she needed a couple of times a week rather than every day. She felt so pleased with the improvement in her health that she had also been motivated to lose weight.

Sandra Herrmann, a practitioner in London, saw a bee keeper who had become severely allergic to bee stings: he would initially become short of breath and then start to choke and have to be hospitalised. After only one HK session in which Sandra worked to remove his allergy, he was stung again and developed severe breathing problems, but this time he found that by the time he reached the hospital his breathing had returned to normal, and he had no need of any further medical treatment.

Correcting Allergies Using The SET Technique

Because it is so powerful, the SET procedure should only be carried out by a skilled HK practitioner. Whereas the tapping technique allows only one substance to be corrected at a time, the SET procedure allows many allergies to be corrected together, providing the energy system gives permission. In HK we always ask for permission from the energy system so that the SET procedure is only used appropriately. Even then it can cause quite a strong reaction in clients. Most practitioners advise clients to drink lots of water for the couple of days following an SET, otherwise headaches and kidney pain can result. Even so, some people still experience a reaction to the SET procedure. The most common one is tiredness, although this usually only lasts at the most for two or three days. See Chapter 9 for more on the SET procedure.

Increasing Tolerance Levels

Tolerance levels are very much affected by stress levels: the more stressed you are, the lower your tolerance to a whole range of substances. So if you are very stressed (e.g. working too hard, arguing with your partner and worrying about money), your tolerance level for everything you eat, drink, inhale, touch, or come into contact with in any way, will be much lower than when you are happy and things are going well in your life. If your tolerance levels are very high in general, you will not notice the effect of a lowering, but if your tolerance levels are already on the low side, this further drop can lead to real problems.

Sometimes the most appropriate way to increase tolerance levels is not by working directly on individual substances, but by working more generally to reduce the client's stress levels. This can be done in one of two ways:

- Identifying specific stresses that need to avoided, such as over work, poor nutrition, and so on

- Strengthening the energy system through corrections, which increase the overall health of the physical body

This will then, usually, lead to an increase in tolerance levels for a whole range of substances, and muscle testing can establish what the new tolerance levels are.

> A client who was recovering from chronic fatigue syndrome had found that in order to stay well she needed to avoid a whole range of different foods, making her diet very restricted and demanding a lot of self-discipline. She came to me because she wanted her allergies fixed. She was rather dubious when, through the muscle testing, I established that we had to work on her body's energy control system (see chapter 6). She phoned me a week later to say that she was now eating normally and feeling great. I suspect that rather than having allergies, she had very low tolerances to a whole range of things and was also extremely sensitive to electromagnetic pollution. By working on her body's energy control system I made her less sensitive to electromagnetic pollution, so that her tolerance levels were able to increase. We did not work directly on allergies or tolerance levels, because her energy system knew that the most effective way to help her was through a different type of energy correction. Her 'allergies' disappeared.

If the person has a problem with one particular substance, or the general work will take some time to have an effect, then the energy system may ask to work directly on improving individual tolerance levels, rather than other factors that would lead to a general rise in tolerance levels. The procedure for increasing tolerance levels to specific substances is very simple. It is similar to the allergy tapping technique, but this time specific points on the body are held while other points are tapped.

There is also an SET tolerance procedure, which can be used instead. As with the SET allergy procedure, this is often used by practitioners in preference to the tapping technique, as it allows many substances to be corrected at the same time.

Once the tolerance tap or the SET tolerance procedure has been carried out the tolerance level will usually increase over a period of time. The practitioner can establish what the new tolerance levels are and give advice to the client on staying within them. The tolerance levels will still go down when the person is stressed, but not as low, and often no further problems will be experienced.

If someone is allergic to something, their tolerance is zero. Once the allergy has been corrected, tolerance levels will often automatically increase, but occasionally the tolerance level remains so low that the client still experiences problems. In these cases the practitioner will carry out the tolerance procedure either immediately after the allergy procedure, or during a subsequent appointment.

Allergy or tolerance work is often combined with other work, depending on what the energy system selects from the menu offered by the practitioner.

> John Payne, a practitioner based in Cornwall, saw a five-year-old child. The mother suspected that the child was reacting to food additives, especially some of

the food colourings. Foods containing food additives seemed to trigger untypical behaviour: the child would be noisy, excited, very contrary and say 'no' very loudly when asked to do anything. As well as correcting the food additive problem with the SET procedure, John had to do some BBEI corrections (see page 67) and a psychological correction (see chapter 7). The mother phoned a month later and told John that from two days after the appointment her daughter had been calmer and there had been no behavioural problems at all. The mother had tried deliberately giving her daughter foods that had previously caused a reaction and even then there had been no problem.

The Use Of HK Allergy Procedures In Conventional Medicine

Unfortunately these simple and effective procedures have not been taken up by many people in the medical profession: they are usually incredulous that such a system can work and dismiss it out of hand without experiencing it. Yet some doctors have put their prejudices aside and investigated it.

A Swiss doctor who has undertaken some HK courses told me that he had been initially sceptical about health kinesiology's claim to be able to correct severe allergic reactions, but, having tried the technique with several patients, he had been impressed by the results. Eventually he decided to use it with patients who had potentially life-threatening anaphylactic reactions to certain foods. In carefully controlled conditions he challenged his patients with the previously highly dangerous foods and found that after the HK treatment they had no adverse reactions. He was extremely impressed by this clear demonstration of health kinesiology's power.

Drugs And Drug Reactions

Drugs and health kinesiology can seem odd bed-fellows, but health kinesiology can help those who are allergic or intolerant to drugs that they need. The same doctor told me that he always uses muscle testing before prescribing an antibiotic to check if the patient will experience an allergic reaction to it. Since he started doing this, he has not had a single patient with an adverse reaction to an antibiotic. He uses the techniques in a simple way. He does not correct an antibiotic allergy, although he knows how to do this, but simply chooses another antibiotic, which is not a problem for the patient.

My experience is that a lot of well-documented side effects to drugs are, in fact, allergy or intolerance reactions. As a health kinesiology practitioner my aim is always to help clients reach a state of health where they do not need any medication, but this is not always possible, or only after a considerable length of time. Using the allergy or intolerance tap or the SET procedure the practitioner can often stop these unpleasant side effects very quickly and make life more tolerable.

A lady with arthritis consulted Josie Donaldson. Not only was she suffering from the effects and pain of the arthritis, but she was also suffering from the side effects of the different tablets that she was taking to help alleviate the arthritis. As well as her arthritis drugs, she was taking aspirin, anti-inflammatory drugs, paracetamol, and was having regular gold injections. She was suffering from heartburn, an acidic stomach, nausea, headaches, weakness of the legs, low blood sugar, and was in chronic pain even with the drugs. Josie found that the client was allergic to some of her drugs and intolerant to others, so she corrected these. By the next appointment all her symptoms apart from the pain had gone. She had no more heartburn, nausea, headaches etc. This inspired her to want to come off the drugs. With the aid of her doctor she was able slowly to wean herself off them, and she is now no longer taking any medication for her arthritis. She has hardly any pain except for odd flare ups, which she controls by using essential oils.

Allergy = Addiction

One of the most fascinating aspects of people's reactions to an allergy is that they often become addicted to the very thing that is causing them problems.

An amusing example of this occurred several years ago when I was visiting a friend. When I went into her kitchen, I discovered cat food scattered all over the floor. She explained that her cat was a messy eater and habitually threw its food around. I was initially surprised at this, because most cats are such fastidious eaters. Remembering that allergy problems can lead to insatiable cravings, I asked if I could test the cat. My testing showed that the cat was allergic to rabbit and turkey: the poor thing was so addicted he was throwing his food around searching for his 'fix'. I corrected his allergies, and he started eating like a normal cat.

People will often really like the thing that they are allergic to, sometimes to the extent that they will crave it and seek it out at any and every opportunity. They will generally not be aware that they are choosing foods that contain the allergen in order to 'feed' their addiction.

Using muscle testing I found that a client was allergic to grapes. She told me that she hardly ever ate grapes, so that could not be her problem. When I questioned her further, she told me that she ate muesli for breakfast (with raisins and sultanas), usually had a salad with a dressing containing wine vinegar for lunch, in the middle of the afternoon she would often have a cup of tea with a piece of fruit cake and then finally she would have a glass of sherry before dinner and a glass of wine with dinner. Raisins, sultanas, wine vinegar, fruit cake, sherry and wine contain grapes in some form or other.

It may seem strange, but smoking is a similar reaction. Many smokers will say that they smoke because it helps them to feel calm and able to face the day. When they first started smoking they did not get this effect from it, because this 'benefit' only occurs as the smoker becomes addicted. If smokers are allergic to tobacco smoke (or the tobacco itself, or the filter or even the paper glue), they are likely to find it extremely difficult to give up. The addiction to the nicotine and the allergy/addiction to some other component of the cigarette reinforce each other.

> Josie Donaldson helped her husband Andy give up smoking, although this was not why he had asked Josie for help. He had injured his knee a month previously and as part of this work an SET allergy correction on tobacco came up. Andy had been smoking since he was fifteen years old. The issue title was *Looking After My Body Better*. Immediately after the session Andy gave up smoking. The next week he became very grumpy and extremely moody and this lasted for about two weeks. Andy said that he was surprised at how easy it was to give up. It has been three years since that treatment: his knees are fine and he does not smoke.

A food that a person is addicted to becomes associated with contentment, happiness and well-being, even though there may be adverse reactions connected with it. The person associates feeling better with the food. When the person does not have the food, irritability and a hunger that is difficult to satisfy result. These symptoms are not associated with the food, because they do not occur when the food is consumed, but occur as the person enters the withdrawal phase of the addiction.

Interestingly small babies often reject foods to which they are allergic, rather than seeking them out. So if a small child steadfastly refuses a food that most children like there are good grounds for suspecting a problem with that food. Unfortunately parents often persist with the food, either by disguising it, or bribing the child to eat it, until the child becomes addicted to it. The child then seeks out the food, and the parents do not usually associate any symptoms the child experiences with the consumption of the allergen.

One explanation for the allergy-addiction phenomenon is that proteins are incompletely digested, as part of the allergic reaction. This produces other substances (peptides) which then act in a similar manner to the body's own peptide hormones. This may stimulate endorphin production in the brain. Endorphins are the body's natural painkillers. The allergy sufferer's body becomes adapted to this elevated level of endorphin activity and craves the substance that maintains this endorphin level.

> One of the first times I used the SET allergy technique was with a client who was showing all the signs of being addicted to her painkillers, which she took in high doses every day. I had been seeing her for some time for the headaches that she had been suffering from for over forty years. These had virtually stopped, but when she tried to cut down on her painkillers she found that she started to shake and feel unwell. She was understandably concerned that she would have to continue with the medication even after the headaches were completely clear. Muscle testing showed that she was allergic to the painkillers. Once the SET procedure was complete she found that she was completely free of her need for them, and her headaches did not return either.

I saw a young teenager who had developed boils inside his nose. Testing showed that he was allergic to correcting fluid. In my naivety I was rather surprised at this, because I assumed he did not use it very often in his schoolwork. He looked very embarrassed and admitted that he had been experimenting with sniffing it. We talked about this, and I did some psychological work on him and corrected his allergy to the correcting fluid. The boils in his nose quickly disappeared and he stopped this potentially dangerous behaviour.

The use of allergy tapping and the SET procedure for drug addiction undoubtedly needs exploring much further.

Unfortunately many people do not realise that the symptoms they are suffering from may be attributable to allergic or intolerance reactions. Even when people do, they often do not know that health kinesiology offers a safe, effective way of counteracting allergies and allowing people to lead more normal lives.

9: Detoxifying The Body

An important part of an HK practitioner's work is enabling the body to detoxify itself. Many books are available which suggest complicated diets or an expensive array of nutritional and herbal supplements for this sort of problem. The HK practitioner has some powerful procedures to do this, so that these other measures may not be needed.

The HK practitioner has three main detoxifying procedures, which work on different aspects of the problem:

- The symbiotic energy transformation (SET) correction - for when the energy system has miscategorized or cannot identify a nutrient or toxic substance.

- The mechanism control correction - for when cell receptor sites have become blocked, and nutrients cannot get into the cell, or toxins cannot be removed.

- The tissue energy block correction - for when the energy is blocked in the tissues, leading to nutrient deprivation or toxic build-up.

Symbiotic Energy Transformation

The SET technique first referred to in chapter 8 can be used in several different situations. As well as correcting allergies, it is also a rapid and effective method of detoxifying the body, enhancing nutrient absorption and supporting psychological change.

The procedure for this correction is very simple: acupuncture points are held or cosmic batteries put in position on the body while the stressor is activated. In an SET this is done by placing various substances, identified through muscle testing, on or near a specific acupuncture point on the body.

The following explanation of the implications of the SET technique has been somewhat simplified for the purposes of this book. Before the physical body can respond to the physical properties of the substance, the body's energy system interacts with the subtle energy properties of the substance. Part of this interaction involves a categorization of the substance, so that the physical body knows what to do with it.

The body has two simple categories:

- This is something I want

- This is something I do not want.

Nutritious foods are categorized as something the body wants, whereas viruses and heavy metals, such as mercury and cadmium, are categorized as things that are not wanted. This is a crucial distinction, because on the basis of it the body mobilizes completely different responses. It does its best to maximize absorption of things it has categorized as wanted and strives to eliminate things it has categorized as not wanted.

What Happens If A Substance Is Miscategorized?

Miscategorization of substances by the energy system is a common problem. When this happens, it means that the physical body attempts to maximize absorption and retention of harmful substances and strives to break down and eliminate substances that are beneficial.

The symbiotic energy technique (SET) is used to correct it. This is the same procedure that was described in the last chapter for allergy corrections. In fact, allergy problems can be seen as a special case of this miscategorization - the body categorizes harmless or even beneficial substances as harmful and produces symptoms such as diarrhoea or a runny nose as a consequence of its attempt to remove the problem substance.

Miscategorizing Toxic Substances

If the energy system miscategorizes a toxic substance, the physical body will not be as efficient at breaking down and excreting the toxic substance, as it would be if it were recognized correctly. In fact, the body may even store the toxin, causing all sorts of problems. The SET correction does not make toxic substances harmless, but it does enable the body to deal with these substances as efficiently as possible.

The SET procedure may be needed for substances that are being regularly encountered or for toxins that were stored in the body years ago.

When I was first introduced to the SET technique my oldest son was eight years old. One of the first things I had to do for him was an SET on general anaesthetics. Jon had had a major operation when he was eight hours old, a minor operation when he was six weeks old and another major operation when he was eighteen months old. Over six years later muscle testing revealed that he needed an anaesthetic detoxification. As a result of this SET, his reading age went up yet again dramatically. (See the introduction for the first occasion this happened.)

If the energy system miscategorizes bacteria or viruses, this makes the body more susceptible to the virus or bacteria. It takes longer to recover and may even develop low-grade infections that become difficult to eradicate using conventional means.

Bernhard Caspar used the SET process to protect several horses from adenitis equorum. This is a highly infectious disease producing a lot of pus, which quickly transfers the disease to other healthy animals. Bernhard found that having applied the appropriate SET procedure, none of the treated horses got the infection, but untreated ones did.

I have had clients come in with a bad cold or the beginnings of flu and walk out sixty minutes later feeling fine. I usually use the SET procedure to help their body quickly recognize and deal with the virus. I have also helped clients with cold sores, genital herpes and shingles. The SET technique teaches the body to recognize the virus at an energy level and deal with it appropriately.

Some years ago I helped a student nurse with psoriasis. Her mother was a client of mine and made an appointment for her daughter, whose psoriasis had flared up because she was about to sit an important examination. It quickly became clear that the daughter was extremely sceptical and had only come to see me because of pressure from her mother. The psoriasis had started after she had a sore throat caused by streptococcal bacteria about five years before. Testing showed that her body had not completely eliminated these bacteria. I used the SET technique to correct the problem, plus some other HK corrections, as determined by muscle testing. Testing indicated that she would notice some benefit within ten days, but that she would need one further appointment to clear the psoriasis completely. The client was clearly deeply incredulous that this could possibly be true, but when she came ten days later her skin was already a lot better. Three weeks later the psoriasis had completely cleared and she sat her exams without further problem. When I next saw the nurse's mother for her own appointment, she gave me a bunch of flowers: "These are from my daughter – she wants to say how sorry she is for being so sceptical and horrible and to thank you for your help."

Miscategorizing Nutrients

As well as miscategorizing toxic substances, the energy system can miscategorize nutrients. If the energy system miscategorizes nutrients, such as calcium or zinc, the body may reject these, and deficiency symptoms may result. Because of the body's inability fully to utilize the substance, much higher levels of the nutrient will be required to meet the body's need. This is one reason why 'normal' levels of a particular vitamin or mineral may be inadequate for some individuals. They will show deficiency signs unless they have an extremely high intake from food, take suitable supplements, or have the problem corrected by a health kinesiologist.

While teaching some practitioners about this problem of nutrient miscategorization, I remarked that white spots on the nails could be a sign of zinc deficiency. One of the practitioners had white spots on her nails, so she decided to check this out. Sure enough, testing showed that her body did not fully recognize zinc as a useful nutrient. She then corrected this. At a conference several months later she rushed up to me, held her finger nails in front of my face and said: "Look!" The top halves of her nails still had the white flecks, but the lower halves were completely free. Since completing the correction her nails were growing without the white flecks, showing that her body had learnt to recognize zinc and use it efficiently.

Cora, a five-year-old female guinea pig started to bite her companion, Lucas, pulling out lots of his long, curly hair. Through muscle testing Bernhard Caspar established that Cora was short of some minerals and was trying to take them in by eating her companion's hair. Bernhard carried out an SET on a series of minerals, provided her with a different diet and the problem disappeared.

I used to assume that, if the body could not absorb a nutrient, it would excrete the excess, but from my HK work with numerous clients I now know that this is not true. It often simply stores the excess inappropriately. It may store it in a way that does not cause any symptoms, or it may store it in a way that does. In the latter situation you may see signs of deficiency and excess within the same body.

Sometimes a miscategorization problem appears to be inherited, although the exact manifestation may vary between family members.

Testing revealed that a client's body did not recognize calcium properly and was putting the excess into her joints and causing arthritis. Her nails were brittle and weak, which is often a sign of calcium deficiency. I explained that she had symptoms of both excess and a deficiency of calcium and that this could be an inherited problem. She immediately told me that her mother had been in hospital recently for tests, and the diagnosis was abnormal levels of calcium around the heart. I never worked on the mother, but it seemed that she too had problems with calcium recognition, but her body dealt with it differently.

Very often testing will show that the client is miscategorizing several substances and some of these can be toxins and some nutrients.

A fifteen-year-old girl with severe epilepsy came to see me. She had been epileptic since the age of seven. In spite of taking the drug epilim, she was still having five to six fits a week. Part of the work I did on her was to help her body to recognize chromium as a nutrient and cadmium as a toxin. Chromium is involved in maintaining correct blood sugar levels, which are vitally important for the brain, and cadmium is a very toxic metal. The SET technique was used, and other HK energy corrections were also required. As a result of her HK treatment she eventually she became fit-free and was able to stop taking the epilim.

A six-year-old boy was brought to see me. He had recently come out of hospital. He had been admitted with suspected meningitis, but nothing had been found. His mother told me that he was always unwell: he vomited frequently, complained of feeling queasy almost every day, produced fatty stools which floated, had a persistent chesty cough, was always tired, pot-bellied, bandy-legged and small for his age. At two years old he had been diagnosed as a coeliac, even though the tests were not positive. Since then he had followed a gluten-free diet. The doctors were now talking about doing tests for cystic fibrosis. When I tested him I found that he was allergic to yeast, soya and airborne moulds, that he was not absorbing three minerals and two amino acids properly, and that his body was not recognizing aluminium as a toxic metal. Further testing indicated that the SET procedure would be the main thrust of the work. When I saw him for the second time a month later his mother told me that he had put on weight, was sleeping better, feeling less sick and was less lethargic. He had grown two centimetres in the month and was now looking forward to being as tall as his father.

Of course, there can be other reasons why a body does not absorb nutrients. For example, if stomach juices are not in the correct acidic balance, digestion does not take place efficiently and effectively. Medication can also affect nutrient absorption by binding with the nutrients so that they cannot be effectively absorbed. Diarrhoea or eating rapidly or under stress can affect nutrient absorption too. These problems will not respond to the SET technique, but HK practitioners have other possibilities for helping in such circumstances.

Miscategorizing Body Chemicals

Sometimes the energy system miscategorizes chemicals produced by the body itself. It is not totally clear what is happening in these situations, but sometimes it seems that one part of the body is busy producing the chemical (for example, a hormone, enzyme or neurotransmitter), and another part of the body is busily trying to destroy it, because it does not recognize it as part of itself. This can result in the body functioning as though it is short of a crucial chemical, even though it is, in fact, producing enough.

At other times the body is not trying to destroy the body chemical but seems unable to correctly respond to the message that it is being given by it. The work I have been doing recently with leptin and other hormones relating to appetite is a new and exciting example of this.

When fat is put into the fat cells, these produce a hormone, leptin. This hormone travels in the blood stream to the hypothalamus (a part of the brain) with a message to reduce the appetite. Fat people generally have high levels of leptin in their blood stream, but it seems that the brain is insensitive to the message, so the fat person goes on eating beyond what is ideal for them. The SET technique has been used very successfully in these situations with amazing results. Within a few days of completing the SET some people find that their appetite has dropped, often dramatically. This happens without any effort on the part of the person: they just feel less hungry, they feel full quicker and at long last feel in control of their appetite. They often also experience a heightened sense of well-being, fewer digestive problems and more energy. Their blood sugar levels are much more stable. They no longer need to diet but lose weight naturally and safely without any struggle and distress. Many clients describe this as a miracle, but it is simply the re-activation of a normal body mechanism.

This works for some over-weight people, but not for all. Even when leptin and other hormones (such as neuropeptides Y, somatostatin, insulin, and so on) are corrected, the appetite remains the same. I am confident that with time we will be able to find the solution for these people too.

"I'm down a dress size"

I came to see Jane because of years of struggling with my weight, having nothing but negative comments from doctors, and being continually bombarded to lose weight. I'm mildly diabetic. I don't overeat, and when I've tried dieting the weight loss has always been minimal and not long term. I used to get very low about it. I read an article Jane had written about bodies' responses and thought it might help.

I felt terrible the day after the first appointment, but then I started to feel great. Six months later and four more appointments and my whole ability to cope with my situation has changed. I won't be made to feel like a second-class citizen by doctors because I'm large – I'm much more confident, much happier about myself. I'm down a dress size – I don't know how much weight I've lost, because I don't weigh myself. I've lost weight without dieting and without it becoming the overall factor running my whole life. In the past I'd go on a diet and that's what would happen – I'd feel bad about myself and it didn't work anyway. My blood sugar is down too. A lot of other hang-ups have disappeared along the way. I'm much more relaxed - my family have noticed a difference. I had been very stiff and not able to do things - lots of little aches and pains – now I'm totally mobile. I'm doing things that I wouldn't have done a year ago. I can't put it in words really. I'm 55, coming up to 56, but I feel I can now hold my own at work and out with my daughter. I feel great.

Client *Pauline Rowe* and Practitioner *Jane Thurnell-Read*

The Use Of Body Samples In An SET

Body samples may be used as part of an SET correction. Saliva, sweat, hair or nail clippings, for example, may be placed on the torso along with the other substances indicated by testing. This almost always strikes clients initially as a strange concept, until I explain further. Saliva may contain enzymes, bacteria and viruses. Urine can contain hormones and metabolic by-products. Earwax may contain metals, drugs or viruses. Eczema and psoriasis scales can be the result of the body's attempt to excrete harmful chemicals, heavy metals or some metabolic by-product it is unable to handle properly. Sometimes the body sample contains beneficial substances that the body has miscategorized and is unable to use properly.

Some years ago I had an upset stomach for a few days. As this got better, I developed acute vertigo. I tested that I should do an SET correction using my earwax. I did this and the vertigo disappeared almost immediately. Interestingly, I have found that most of the people I see with vertigo need an SET on their earwax as part of their treatment.

One of my sons had a friend to play. The friend had received a TB vaccination some weeks before, but the vaccination site was still oozing and weeping and causing him considerable pain and distress. I asked his mother if I could help him. She agreed, and I carried out the SET procedure, using the discharge from his arm. I saw his mother about a week later and she said: "I don't know what you did, but it certainly did the trick."

If the body stores the wrongly categorized substance in the hair or the nails, this will often result in their structure being disturbed so that they break easily. After the SET, the health of the hair or nails often improves dramatically, and this can be a welcome side effect of a health kinesiology treatment.

Sometimes the energy system wants to eliminate something, such as a drug or virus, which is not accessible through the usual body samples. If the substance is locked deep in some cells, the practitioner may be able to do corrections, which bring it to a more accessible place, for example, the bloodstream.

When I met my partner, John Payne, he had recurring bouts of illness characterized by sudden high temperatures and total prostration. This situation would occur every few months and last for several days. We decided to see if we could correct this problem using HK. During the first session it became clear that John was suffering from a recurring viral infection and that the virus would 'hide' in his body between the attacks. The work of this first session was to bring the virus into the blood stream so that it could be worked on. The energy system indicated that once this work had been done, it would take some time before the virus was in the blood stream. In fact, the body was extremely precise: the next session had to take place between 20th and 24th December. We meant to make a note in the diary, but did not, and so we forgot all about it. By 26th December John was feeling extremely unwell. Suddenly I remembered about the work we had to do, and we very quickly completed the SET on the blood. Unfortunately, by now the virus was well entrenched in the bloodstream and it took John almost three weeks to become well again. The body had been so specific about the date for the session, because it recognized that between 20th and 24th December, the virus would be in the bloodstream making it available for the HK work, but not in such proportions that it would cause symptoms. We both learnt a valuable lesson from this unfortunate experience, but fortunately since that time (five to six years ago) John has not had any recurrence of the symptoms.

Test Kits

Sometimes it is not possible to use a body sample for a correction. The hormone, enzyme, virus or bacteria may not be readily available from a body sample, even if preliminary work is carried out. In other cases the substance may be present, but a body sample would contain other things that the energy system is not ready to have corrected.

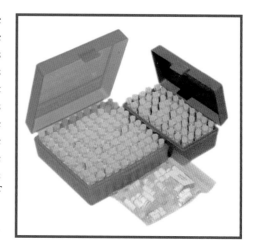

Test kits

In these situations a sample of the specific substance must be used. As it is the energy pattern that the practitioner is correcting rather than the physical properties of the substance, this may be in homeopathic form. This allows practitioners to have access to safe and convenient samples of otherwise hazardous, unstable, expensive or rare substances. A range of test samples is available for this purpose. These are glass vials containing homeopathic versions of hormones, enzymes, neuro-transmitters, amino acids, viruses, bacteria and so on. This is such an important part of HK that much of my time in recent years has been spent researching and tracking down substances for test kits.

At one point I had a problem with bleeding gums, so when I read about some new research into the role of an enzyme, cathepsin C, in preventing periodontal disease and gingivitis, I decided to obtain a sample of cathepsin C for testing. Testing showed that my energy system did not recognize cathepsin C, hence my bleeding gums. I carried out the SET correction and by the very next day my gums had stopped bleeding. I told some HK practitioners about this. Josie Donaldson was interested because her cat, Zippy, had gingivitis. She obtained a test vial of the enzyme from me and used it in an SET for Zippy, and her gingivitis cleared up completely.

Using Flower Essences And Homeopathic Remedies In An SET

Flower remedies and homeopathic remedies are traditionally taken orally (see page 138), but health kinesiology practitioners have another rather novel way of using them. They can be used as part or as the whole of an SET. This is equivalent to the person taking the remedy. As well as enhancing physical well-being, homeopathic and flower remedies used in this way can help clients to become happier, more confident and more optimistic – just as they would if taken orally. Muscle testing establishes exactly which remedies are needed, and whether they should be taken in the traditional way or used in an SET.

Sara Gibbons of Harrogate saw a client who had given up her job temporarily because of other stresses in her life. She was suffering from extreme fatigue and rhinitis. By the second visit she was already beginning to feel better in herself and had more energy. The client talked to Sara about the problems she was experiencing in her private life. After this Sara found her body simply wanted an SET with Bach Flower Remedies. The client was amazed at the appropriateness of the remedies that her energy system had chosen by muscle testing, particularly as Sara had tested them without looking at the labels on the bottles. On the next session the client reported significant increases in energy levels and an ability to deal with stressful situations more easily.

SET Reactions

The SET procedure is a very powerful detoxifying procedure and in consequence sometimes causes strong reactions. The most common ones are:

- Extreme tiredness

- Thirst

- Existing symptoms temporarily becoming worse

- Excessive sweating

- More frequent urination

- Diarrhoea

- Flu-like symptoms

These reactions usually last no more than one or two days, and some people do not experience any adverse reaction at all. Drinking extra water for a few days may aid the detoxifying process and minimize the chances of uncomfortable reactions.

Mechanism Control

Mechanism control corrections are part of the energy control system corrections group, but as they are involved in detoxifying the body it is more appropriate to cover them here. These corrections are used to unblock cell receptor sites. If a cell receptor site is blocked, nutrients cannot get into and toxins cannot get out of the cell. This is different from the body not recognizing the substance, and so is dealt with differently, using mechanism control corrections.

Cell receptor sites are specific and only allow certain substances – ones needed by the cell – to enter. A simple but effective analogy is that of a toy that has several differently shaped holes, through which the correctly shaped pieces have to be posted.

If the receptor site is occupied by another substance, such as a drug or a toxic metal, nutrients cannot get in. There may be an adequate supply of the nutrient, but the cells in a particular organ or tissue are unable to utilize it if the receptor site is blocked. In order for the cell to have access to the nutrient the cell receptor site has to be unblocked. This is the job of mechanism control corrections.

Cells can be seen as small factories, and as part of their activity they produce waste – metabolic by-products. The body needs to be able to remove these from the cells to avoid a toxic build up. Cell receptor sites are involved in this process, and if they are blocked, the cell is unable to remove this waste matter. Mechanism control corrections can resolve this problem.

For mechanism control corrections, the energy system is rebalanced, while the stress is activated by the client actually carrying out instructions, so as to generate specific feelings, experiences or sensations. Typical instructions to the client are *feel relaxed* or *experience trust* or *accept change* or *know that you can love others*. It is not known why doing corrections in this way unblocks cell receptor sites, but this is what happens.

Some clients need both mechanism control corrections and the SET procedure.

One client in his forties had received high doses of antibiotics as a small child. Through muscle testing we established that some of this antibiotic was still in his body and was blocking cell receptor sites of the optic nerve. We also discovered that his body did not recognize the energy pattern of the antibiotic and would not know what to do with it even if it were released from the cell receptor sites, so the work was carried out in two stages, a week apart. In the first session a mechanism control correction removed the antibiotic from the cell receptor sites and, in the second session, an SET procedure allowed the body to dispose of the antibiotic once it had been freed.

After the first session I told the client he might experience a lot of earwax over the next week. (I had established through muscle testing that we would be using earwax for the SET). He was somewhat taken aback by this and said that he had never had any problems with earwax and could not see why he would do so now. I explained that I had carried out a correction to get the antibiotic out of the cell receptor sites, but because the body did not recognize the antibiotic properly, it would try to dispose of it inappropriately through his earwax.

He was very sceptical but agreed not to clean his ears, if his body did start to produce excessive amounts of earwax. When he came back for the second session, he told me that his body had indeed produced a lot of earwax during the intervening week. We were able to use the earwax as part of an SET correction.

Tissue Energy Blocks

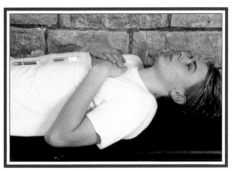

A tissue energy block with the cosmic batteries in place

As the name suggests, tissue energy block corrections (TEBs) resolve problems with energy blocks in the tissues. These blocks are often caused by injury or sudden movements, and will hamper the flow of nutrients into and the removal of toxins from those tissues.

For TEB corrections, acupuncture points are held or cosmic batteries are placed on the client's body, whilst the stress is activated – in this case by placing the client's hands on their body. Sometimes it is clear why the hands are in a particular place, but not always.

TEBs can help people in many ways: pain and discomfort can disappear, and people can feel better psychologically too.

A client, who had suffered with severe agoraphobia for seventeen years, needed work involving a lot of TEBs on her neck. Some time later she told me that she had been born with the umbilical cord around her neck and nearly died. I am certain that this traumatic event created energy disturbances around her neck. The agoraphobia had started when her first child was born. I think that the birth of her child triggered some deep, subconscious memories of her own birth and struggle for breath. It took several years of HK work, but eventually she made a full recovery.

Practitioner Kathy Bradley had a client who needed tissue energy blocks. The client had to put her hands on her face. She was extremely impressed by this, because she had an extremely painful tooth abscess exactly where the hands were placed. She had not told Kathy about this. The abscess quickly disappeared, much to the client's delight.

Sometimes the results of TEB corrections can be dramatic and unexpected.

Practitioner Sue Palmer saw a middle-aged lady who had suffered a mild stroke in 1980 affecting the right side of the brain. Since that time she had suffered balance difficulties and vertigo. She found it difficult looking down, for example over bridges. She had difficulty walking down slopes, because she felt as if she would fall. She also felt carsick if she looked down whilst the car moved. Sue did two mechanism control corrections followed by two tissue energy block items – both on the forehead. Immediately after the correction, the client said it was the exact location where she had been hit by an iron bar at the age of ten. One month later her balance was much better, she was able to read in a car without feeling sick and she had walked down a very steep slope with only a little support from her partner, who was amazed.

Amanda Brooks used tissue energy blocks in less than ideal circumstances. She got talking to an old lady in a park. The lady had very painful legs with a lot of fluid retention around the ankles. She could only walk a hundred yards before it became too painful to go on. Amanda did not have any of her equipment with her, but nevertheless she offered to help. Amanda completed tissue energy blocks on the back of the woman's right calf as indicated by muscle testing. The lady looked as though she was just humouring Amanda, but afterwards she phoned and said that she had walked half a mile with no pain that very day. This improvement was still evident eighteen months later.

Each of these three different types of energy correction (SET, mechanism control and tissue energy blocks) works in a different way to improve the function of the physical body by removing toxins and increasing nutrient absorption. When the physical body is functioning more efficiently, people will often feel better psychologically too. It is no wonder that these corrections are considered to be so powerful.

Practitioner Rob Adams saw seven-year-old Matthew Sergison. Matthew has cerebral palsy and is not capable of any control or speech. In the first session tissue energy block corrections were carried out and in the second session a BBEI *fear that I won't be understood* came up. In the following week Matthew smiled for the first time in his life.

10: Energy Flow Balancing

Energy flow balancing (EFB) corrections are concerned with helping the body to function more efficiently given the structure it has. Because energy flow balancing corrections are concerned with function rather than structure, the changes will often happen very rapidly. Structural changes often need time for healing and repair to take place, but functional changes can often take place instantly once the energy conflict has been resolved. Many clients will notice the benefit of energy flow balancing corrections the same day that the corrections are done.

No more medication

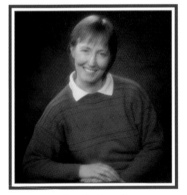

Sandie Lovell

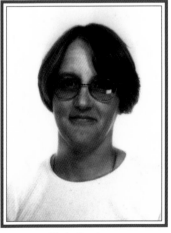

Chris Pattinson

When Chris Pattinson came to see me, she was suffering from rheumatoid arthritis, fibromyalgia, asthma and early menopause. She was taking a cocktail of different drugs to control her symptoms but was unhappy with all the side effects. Four weeks after our first session she phoned to inform me that her fibromyalgia symptoms had gone – stiff hips and 'wobbly legs'. Chris was delighted.

Her body requested long gaps between sessions, so the treatment took place over some months. We covered several issues including energy flow in the skeletal, immune, endocrine, digestive and excretory systems, and the secretion of chemicals/hormones. On a psychological level we dealt with her self appreciation.

When there are particular stressful periods in her life her 'wobbly legs' due to the fibromyalgia start to re-appear, but a session of HK soon returns her to a state of well-being. Her arthritis is improving, to the point that when she had her wrists X-rayed her consultant was amazed to see that her joints were going back to normal. She no longer needs to take any medication.

Client *Chris Pattinson* and Practitioner *Sandie Lovell*

A discussion of the full range of energy flow balancing corrections is beyond the scope of this book, and this chapter covers only some of the possibilities. (Another type of EFB correction, body position memory, is discussed on page 128.)

Many EFB corrections are concerned either with how the physical senses process information or with how the brain interprets that information. These corrections do not change structure, but they ensure that the physical senses are functioning optimally. For example, energy flow balancing corrections will not correct a squint, because this is caused by structural problems (a fault in the development of the mechanism for aligning the eyes), but will ensure that the eyes function as well as they can and with the minimum amount of stress, given the existing physical constraints.

> A student with severe hearing problems volunteered for a class EFB demonstration. At the end of the day he told me that he was not hearing any better, but, for the first time that he could remember, he did not have a headache and neck pains, which were the usual occurrence after spending most of the day with other people. The energy flow balancing correction had helped to remove some of the stress from his situation, so that the headache and neck pain did not develop. He was overwhelmed by this improvement and had difficulty expressing his gratitude to me.

If there are severe structural problems, EFB work will be able to improve functioning up to a certain level that is constrained by the structural problems. However, even without structural problems, most people are not functioning optimally, so EFB corrections can help to make everyday tasks and experiences easier and less stressful. EFB corrections can help to improve sensory perception or intellectual functioning, so that, for example, night driving is less difficult, or organizing paperwork becomes easier, or studying becomes less stressful. EFB corrections also have a lot to offer people who want to excel in sport or creative activity - the possibilities are endless.

The Basic EFB Correction Procedure

Energy flow balancing corrections follow the same basic procedure as other corrections: the practitioner identifies the stressor, triggers the stress in a controlled manner and either holds acupuncture points or places cosmic batteries on the client's body to rebalance the system.

Each type of correction uses a different way of triggering the stress: for psychological corrections the client has to think something, for allergy corrections substances are placed on the client's body, for tissue energy blocks the client has to place their hands on their body, and for mechanism control corrections the person has to generate sensations within the body. For EFB corrections the client has to **perform** the stressful task. It is not enough to think about it, because this does not activate the required neural pathways. If the client has difficulty hearing monotonous voices, the practitioner sets up a task involving listening to monotonous voices. If the client finds it difficult to turn their head to the right, this is the task they are given. (The precise detail is always carefully tested, to avoid the possibility of injury or unnecessary discomfort.)

> Jayne Walker helped a client who was having vision problems while driving. She told Jayne that if she looked into the far distance while driving, she sometimes experienced 'dizziness and something like migraine in the eyes'. This was happening more frequently and the client was beginning to become concerned. It also happened occasionally in supermarkets, when she looked up at a high shelf. Two EFB corrections came up. The first involved her looking up and down, but with her head tilted slightly upwards. The second involved her standing at a window, looking across the street, and then back at the wood of the window frame, and then across the street again: in other words a repeated change of focus from far to near. This sequence was repeated until the correction was complete. The client was very relieved that this simple treatment stopped the problem completely.

If the client finds the task extremely difficult, this is not a sign that the practitioner has found the wrong task, but an indication that it is exactly right. As the correction takes place the client will usually find the task progressively easier to do; the body will often relax, and the look of strained concentration on the client's face will disappear.

> A client asked me if I could help her dog, because the dog did not like going for a walk! The dog was, rather inappropriately in the circumstances, called Flash. His owner explained that when he heard the sound of his lead he would take no notice and would continually sit down when she tried to take him for walks. In other respects he was a normal, healthy dog. Testing showed he needed some EFB corrections in the sub-category 'kinesthetic'. To put it more simply, he was stressed by walking! The correction took a long time to complete because Flash repeatedly sat down, and his owner would have to haul him to his feet by pulling strenuously on his lead to make him continue walking - it was a hilarious session. The end result was a normal dog - eager to go for a walk at any and every opportunity.

Sometimes the stressful activity has to be performed in its entirety, but in some cases it is enough to isolate the critical components and set these up for the correction. This makes it possible to help people involved in active sports. For example, instead of getting the client to play squash in the practitioner's office, it may be sufficient to correct stresses concerning the position of the hand on the racket, moving quickly sideways, rotating the shoulder through part of its range, and so on.

Sensory Energy Functioning Corrections

A major sub-category of EFB corrections is called sensory energy functioning (SEF) – the three examples used in this chapter so far fit into this category. SEF is concerned with making sure that physical sensory information is transmitted to the brain as effectively as possible. SEF problems often involve the eyes, the ears or a particular body position or movement. Other possibilities include the senses of smell and taste, and the sensation of touching or being touched.

> Sue Davies had problems with her right knee. Two operations had helped, but when she started to do yoga the right knee would hurt the evening afterwards and for a couple more days. Sue was really enjoying the yoga class and was reluctant to give it up. There were three separate EFB items to do: lying down, standing up normally and standing up but with her knees bent. Two days later her knee was very swollen and very painful and she had difficulty walking. She went to bed feeling she would not be able to walk at all the next day, and was surprised when she woke the next morning, and it was a little better. It gradually improved after that, and now she has no problems with her knees.

Whenever I read about someone killing a baby because it would not stop crying, I wonder if an EFB correction for the sound of a baby crying carried out on the person responsible might possibly have averted a dreadful tragedy.

> Some years ago a woman came to see me with her small baby, who had eczema. At one point the baby started crying, and the mother immediately became very agitated. Unable to calm her down, I stopped working on the baby and asked if I could check her out. Sure enough she needed an EFB correction for the sound of a baby crying. We completed the correction – she had to listen to her baby crying. A few weeks later at another appointment for the baby, she told me that I had transformed her life. Now, when the baby cried, she did not get upset and confused, but could think about the problem logically and decide what needed to be done.

If the client knows what the problem is, the practitioner will usually only need to muscle test a few questions to establish the necessary task or tasks.

> A client with a passion for golf told me that her handicap had not improved for some time: she had won the annual golf club booby prize for the last two years! Testing showed that various positions in the golf swing were stressful, so she held one of her golf clubs and I tested to find the exact positions. Each one was corrected, and afterwards she said: "If this works, I'm not telling anyone, as they'll all come to see you, and then I'll be back at the bottom again." Her golf did improve and, true to her word, she did not tell a soul.

Cognitive Sensory Energy Integration

There is another EFB subcategory called cognitive sensory energy integration (CSEI), which is concerned with how the brain interprets the information it receives. This may sound complicated, but the example of reading difficulties should make it clearer. There are many different reasons for problems with reading, but within the EFB category there are two distinct possibilities.

First, the markings on the paper may not be transmitted correctly to the brain. For example, the person may experience stress looking at black on a white background, or when tracking their eyes from left to right. This is a sensory energy functioning problem, and to correct it, the practitioner sets up a task involving the problem skill.

Second, the reading problem could be caused by a difficulty in interpreting the information within the brain, even though it has been correctly received. This is a cognitive sensory energy integration problem, so the appropriate task is one that stimulates this part of the reading process.

It is, of course, possible to have both problems. In this case both sensory energy functioning corrections and cognitive sensory energy integration corrections are needed.

A wide range of functions can be improved by cognitive sensory energy integration corrections. They can help to improve the ability to think systematically, logically, rationally or creatively. If a client is not very good at problem-solving or evaluating information, CSEI corrections may be called for. These corrections can help everyone, because thinking and learning are an integral part of life.

Memory Problems

Although poor memory can be due to physical failings, it can also be a result of CSEI stresses. If CSEI corrections for remembering come up, it means there is either a problem laying down new memories, or a problem retrieving existing memories.

For laying down new memories, the task for the correction will involve trying to remember something new. For retrieving memories, the task will be to remember something from the past. The exact detail is established through muscle testing.

Some people only have problems remembering particular types of information. They may, for example, be able to remember faces, but be completely unable to remember telephone numbers. Some people remember best if they **see** something visually; others remember best if they **hear** something. So, as well as establishing whether the task involves laying down or retrieving memories, the practitioner also has to find out if the memories need to be of a particular type.

I used to find it impossible to remember directions given to me when I was in an unfamiliar area. I would be able to retain the first two or three parts of the directions, but when I had completed those, I would have to stop and ask again. I used to become very exasperated with myself that I could not remember the full sequence of directions I had been given. Eventually I carried out a CSEI correction on myself for remembering directions (laying down sequential auditory information). This is a small thing, but, when I am lost, it reduces the stress immensely knowing that I will be able to remember all the directions given to me.

Correcting these sorts of problems makes life both easier and more pleasurable, allowing greater retention of useful or interesting information and experiences.

"For the first time in my life it was really easy."

Once, when I was a student practitioner, we were practicing energy flow balancing corrections. What came up for me was to look to the left whilst keeping my face facing straight ahead. I was a bit surprised to find that it actually hurt my left eye to do this. When the correction was done, I didn't really think about it that much.

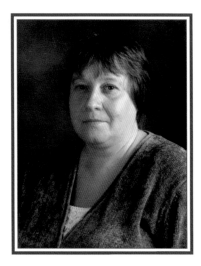

The following week I'd been to an exercise class and I was about to drive home. Normally I drive the long way round because it's so difficult to turn the car around there. This time, for some reason, I spotted a tiny side street and decided to try reversing into it.

The street I was in was full of parked cars on both sides, as was the side street. Normally I wouldn't dream of reversing in such a confined space with so many cars around. This time I just went for it. And it was easy! I couldn't believe it. For the first time in my life it was really easy.

Then I realised why. I was now able to twist a long way round to my left which meant, for a change, I could actually see where I was going. Suddenly I realised why other people were much more confident than me at reversing a car. It wasn't because they were better drivers. It was simply because they could see where they were going. And now I could too.

I sent a card to the other student saying "Thanks! The streets of Hackney are a safer place!"

A bonus to this is that stiffness and pain in my left shoulder has gone. Now I could see (because it wasn't happening any more) that the real problem had been that it hurt my left eye to look to the left, so my body stiffened to stop me going any further to the left. Now the stiffness in my left shoulder has gone, along with pain in my back by the left shoulder blade, and my whole posture is realigning.

Sally Ann Smith

Improving Understanding

The ability to understand can be improved using CSEI corrections. Sometimes the problem is in understanding a particular **type** of information; technical information may be easy to understand, but abstract information may be difficult, or vice versa. Information presented visually may help some, but not others. Some people find they understand things better if they watch a demonstration; others learn better if they are told what to do, and others learn best by doing. EFB corrections can make it easier to understand information that is presented in a way that the client had previously found difficult.

Focusing On More Than One Thing At Once

Sometimes people have difficulty focussing on two things at the same time. For example, having to write and listen at the same time causes stress for many students. Moving sideways while keeping track of a tennis ball may be a problem for an amateur tennis player. Speaking and doing something at the same time can be stressful for a parent trying to answer children's questions and cook the dinner. In these and many other similar situations, the practitioner finds two tasks that the client has to try to do with equal attention while the correction is carried out.

Attention And Distraction

Sometimes the problem is not that two tasks have to be done simultaneously, but that one has to be done with attention, while something else is ignored. In each case muscle testing is used to establish an appropriate focus of attention, and the distraction to trigger the stress while the correction is carried out.

For example, a driver needs to be able to concentrate on the road ahead and ignore the movements of someone sitting in the passenger seat. If concentrating on what someone is saying while there is a background noise is a problem, the CSEI correction will involve the client listening to what is said while a background noise is generated. Testing will establish whether the **type** of background noise is important, e.g. people talking, traffic noise, and so on.

This sort of correction can be particularly useful for hyperactive children and those with attention-deficit disorder. Hyperactive children are often unable to ignore things, so a new sight or sound is not kept in the background, but instantly becomes the focus of attention. Even small noises are sources of distraction, as are such things as the sight of a cat through the classroom window. These corrections can be equally applicable for anyone trying to concentrate while working in a busy, noisy environment.

Some people have the opposite problem: they become so engrossed in something that they are completely oblivious to everything else. This can be an extremely valuable trait, but in some situations it can be at best anti-social, and at worst potentially very dangerous. A parent at home with children has to be able to concentrate on the task in hand, while also being aware of the background noise of the children.

Learning

The ability to learn can be dramatically improved by EFB corrections. Corrections for remembering, understanding and being able to think logically and systematically may be important here, as may psychological corrections concerned with being successful.

Corrections for specific physical skills may also be important if the student is to succeed.

Amanda Brooks saw a client who was studying for a degree course in art & design. Six months into the course she was far behind in the work and found that she was unable to draw anything! She felt physically sick, scared and had panic attacks whenever she picked up a pencil or even thought about it. She had been to Amanda for other problems so did not hesitate to ask for more help. Amanda did four EFB corrections: holding a pencil, looking at a blank piece of paper, putting pencil to paper, and the final item was actually drawing. Amanda also gave the client some earth energy drops to take. (These are similar to Bach flower remedies). The client noticed the improvement within one week and went on successfully to complete her degree. She subsequently wrote to Amanda: " Without your knowledge, understanding and insight I am quite certain that I would have ended up in a mental hospital."

"The day after the session he sat down and did his homework without any fuss"

Jacob was ten years old when he came to see me. He had been diagnosed with mild specific learning disabilities. He was experiencing difficulties at school and couldn't read his own handwriting without pointing at every word. In the first session we did an energy flow balancing correction – he had to read a boring piece out of a newspaper, which he was reluctant to do. His reading so improved after this that both Jacob and his mother were amazed. We also did a body position memory correction – he had to sit at the kitchen table. Jacob complained that it really hurt to sit like that, but he did it so that the stress from sitting in that position could be removed. Before the appointment his mother had endured months of screaming matches over Jacob doing his homework, but the day after the session with me he sat down and did his homework without any fuss. Jacob himself said that his reading was no longer a problem and his mother commented that he has a more positive attitude both generally and towards his homework. His confidence and faith in himself have also increased.

Client "*Jacob*" and Practitioner *Donna Feldman*

Sports Performance

The HK practitioner can help improve sports performance dramatically, and EFBs are often involved. Hand-eye coordination corrections can help tennis, badminton and cricket players. Foot-eye coordination corrections can help footballers. Corrections for a particular body position or movement can help improve performance in many different sports.

Lorrie Duffy helped a teenage boy who was having difficulty with his skateboarding. Whenever he tried to do a jump from the board and then place his feet back on the board, he was unable to do it. Lorrie found out through testing that in his rapid body growth as a teenager some confusion had arisen as to where his feet were! Lorrie completed three energy flow balancing corrections. He put the corrections to the test three weeks later and found he was able to do the jumps without any problem.

As well as helping sportspeople to perform better, EFB corrections can also help them to avoid injury.

Some years ago I took part in a five-day 250-mile (400 km) cycle ride through Cuba. By the third or fourth day one of the teenagers was beginning to develop pain in his knees. He accepted my offer of help. Using muscle testing I established that there were particular points in the cycling action where the angle of his knee caused him problems. He sat on his bicycle, held up by some of the other young men, and I tested for the exact positions. He then had to hold each position in turn while I held the relevant acupuncture points. The rider and the other young men were clearly fascinated, but a little sceptical that this 'weird approach' could possibly work. However, later the same day the young cyclist told me his knees had rapidly improved, and he was now pain free.

Physical And Mental Handicap

HK can often help those who are physically handicapped or who have a genetic condition, by helping these people to function at one hundred per cent of their capability, whatever that capability is.

Pat Ward started to see James when he was fifteen months old. He was diagnosed as having anhidrotic ectodermal dysplasia (an inability to sweat and therefore lack of body temperature control; growing very few, mostly deformed teeth; very sparse hair; skin problems and choking on food because saliva is not produced). Before AED was diagnosed formally, Pat had already helped him with the choking problem. Two EFB corrections were needed: for one he had to eat biscuits, and for another he had to put his fingers in jelly. The choking problem disappeared in a couple of days and he also started to touch his food, something that he had previously refused to do at all. Much to the doctors' amazement, there are traces of sweat now; his hair is getting thicker and his breathing has stopped being a problem. Because of all his problems, James developed a real fear of doctors and hospitals. This fear disappeared over night after Pat worked on him, and he is now quite happy to go and see any doctor. Last time he went to the hospital he said to his mother afterwards: "Go and see Pat now."

Some years ago a Down's syndrome child who was about six years old was brought to see me. His mother said that what she wanted most was for his language skills to improve. She explained that his sentences were only one or two words long and they both got very frustrated and stressed by his inability to communicate his needs. I explained that it was extremely unlikely that I could give her son the speech abilities of a normal six-year-old, but that we could work to ensure he was achieving his language potential, whatever that was. When she came back for his next appointment, she told me that he was now speaking regularly in three to five word sentences. He had even managed one six-word sentence - "Oh dear, I've wet my pants".

EFB And Psychological Problems And Corrections

Sometimes problems appear to be psychological, but muscle testing reveals them to be entirely or largely EFB problems. Fortunately the HK practitioner does not have to guess what is going on: muscle testing provides the means of establishing exactly what is needed.

Practitioner Klaus Schäfer told me how he helped a client who had a strong fear of being with a lot of people, at a conference or in a big department store, for example. Klaus carried out two EFB corrections involving hearing, and one other correction. When the client came for his next appointment, he reported that the pain in his ears had disappeared. Klaus knew nothing about this pain, because the client failed to mention it during his first appointment. He also told Klaus that he had been to a conference and out shopping several times after the first appointment – the first time in more than two years.

However, sometimes a problem that seems likely to respond to energy flow balancing corrections needs psychological ones instead.

A keen badminton player asked me if I could help her improve her game. I had already treated her successfully for a physical problem, so she knew the power of health kinesiology. When we discussed the problem before the session I assumed I would be doing a lot of EFB work, but muscle testing pinpointed a different problem: she took pity on her opponents when she started to win, and subconsciously she then started to make mistakes, so that she ended up losing. A few simple psychological corrections were all that were needed to improve her game.

These examples demonstrate the enormous power of HK muscle testing. It may seem obvious that a certain type of work is right, but the energy system knows what is needed. Muscle testing ensures that the appropriate treatment for the client's unique situation is accurately and quickly discovered.

Energy flow balancing corrections produce a fascinating diversity of procedures, although all follow the same standard pattern of the client performing a stressful task while the system is rebalanced.

EFB corrections can make everyday tasks easier to accomplish; they can help people to perform better at work and in their hobbies and sport; they can help anyone to live up to their true potential.

"Her life is improving"

My sister contracted meningitis as a baby, which resulted in her being partially brain damaged. She is 40 years old this year, but mentally has the age of a young teenager. This has brought about several problems affecting her quality of life. Although through the years she has received a lot of care and attention and there has been improvement since childhood, there are still a number of things that could be changed.

Tracy has suffered from an intolerable amount of fear and stress in her workplace and home life, over things that may seem rather trivial to other people. Such were the overwhelming feelings, she would suffer from migraines that would leave her bedridden for days and she would lose a considerable amount of weight. This had a knock on effect for my mother (whom she still lives with). The meningitis also left her with poor co-ordination and balance and she has fallen at work on several occasions resulting in back injuries. Tracy suffered from several food allergies, which brought on painful headaches. She also got menstrual headaches and cramps, had low confidence and often experienced a feeling of general unhappiness.

Since doing regular sessions with Tracy, she no longer suffers from a great deal of stress at work and doesn't return home with the headaches. She is a lot more confident than she has ever been. A lot of the food allergies have been cleared, and she is able to enjoy more of her favourite foods without consequence. Her appetite has increased and she has actually gained weight for the first time in years. Her menstrual headaches have decreased and her cramps have ceased. Her complexion has greatly improved.

I'm currently working on her balance and co-ordination - Tracy has already noticed a slight improvement - and I hope to work on her writing skills in the future. There's just so much HK can do to help her and it's really rewarding for us all to watch her develop and see how her life is improving.

Client *Tracy Shields* and Practitioner *Je-An Shields*

11: Emergencies, Accidents, Operations, And Scars

It may be thought that complementary therapies can only help with chronic problems, and that for acute problems either drugs or surgery are needed. This is certainly not the experience of HK practitioners. HK has been used very successfully in emergency situations and to help counteract the effects of operations, drugs and the trauma of accidents.

Accidents And Emergencies

Accidents can have a profound and lasting effect on people. Health kinesiology practitioners and students can often recount how they have helped someone's bones to knit faster or damaged organs to regain their former strength. Obviously, if it is a medical emergency, it is essential to contact the medical authorities too.

> Practitioner Briony Latham was phoned by a very distressed client, who had just had boiling water poured on to her thigh. She came to see Briony immediately, and only one correction was needed. Fresh, raw potato also had to be put on the burnt area to help alleviate the symptoms. Two days later there was hardly any sign of the burn, which she said had in fact been a relatively painless experience after the treatment.

> A client phoned to tell me that her husband was suffering from severe abdominal pain. His GP had said that his appendix might need to be removed, but they would have to wait a little longer to be sure. My client knew HK was very good in situations where people are experiencing pain, and she asked me if I could help him. I told her that I would be happy to see him, but that his energy system probably would not give permission for us to remove the pain if surgery were important. Testing showed that he was allergic to some new paint he was using in his work, so we corrected that and his pain completely disappeared and did not return, and he did not need an appendix operation.

Although most HK practitioners will use a lot of equipment, such as magnets, cosmic batteries and test kits, it is possible to manage with the minimum of equipment if necessary. Because of this, HK is a suitable therapy for many first-aid situations.

> Some years ago I was teaching in Russia and was having lunch in the restaurant we used most of the time. The owner approached me because a bee had stung one of his staff. The man's whole arm was swelling as a result. The hospitals were in such a poor state at that time that the man felt it was not worth going to one, so they decided to ask me for help instead. I had no equipment with me, and had to improvise, ending up doing the session in the kitchen using the leaf of a plant as my only equipment. Muscle testing had shown that something green needed to be placed on his arm: a plant in the kitchen happened to be the correct shade. His arm

improved rapidly and at our farewell dinner the proprietor presented me with a bottle of vodka in appreciation of my help.

On the bike ride through Cuba mentioned on page 123, I provided various cyclists with emergency help. I had taken hardly any equipment with me, because I expected to be concentrating on the cycling, but very quickly I found my services in demand. The first person I worked on was a pharmaceutical laboratory representative. He had injured his knee skiing three weeks earlier, and the long plane journey had made the problem much worse – he could not bend his knee at all. He was sure he was not going to be able to ride and was extremely unhappy at this thought. I tentatively offered to do some HK on him and he readily accepted. By the next morning he could bend his knee, was virtually pain free and was able to ride his bike the forty miles planned for that day with the minimum of discomfort. He told everyone what had happened, and soon I had a regular 'clientele' of people seeking help for sore knees and shoulders, allergic reactions to insect bites, headaches, etc. With a few further mini-sessions the salesman completed the whole bike ride easily.

A GP on the ride asked me for help with her swollen knee: she had been unable to ride and had been travelling in the support vehicle because of the pain. Immediately after the treatment she decided to ride again and completed the rest of the ride without any trouble. On one day this included riding a very steep and arduous road to our hilltop stopover point.

Many of the 'consultations' were on the grass verge during a break for water and were often only ten to twenty minutes long, but even so my success rate was high.

Body Position Memory Corrections

Body position memory corrections are a type of energy flow balancing corrections (see chapter 10). They often come up as a result of accidents. When a traumatic event happens, it can be 'stored' in the body in such a way that the energy system associates that particular body position with stress and trauma.

For a body position memory correction each part of the body has to be placed in the exact physical position that will trigger the stress. Interestingly, there is often a point at which the client spontaneously puts themselves into the rest of the position once the practitioner has placed part of the body. Once the client is in the correct position the practitioner will hold acupuncture points or place cosmic batteries on the client. This procedure removes the physical stress associated with the position and can also lead to the release of emotional stress too.

Briony Latham carried out a body position memory correction for a client who had been in a serious car accident a few years previously. Since the accident the client had woken each morning with a stiff, sore neck. The correction had to be done with her in the position in which she was found. She was unconscious after the accident, and so had no conscious memory of anything. After careful muscle testing,

Briony put her in a very precise position: on her right side, with arms and legs and hands carefully positioned and with her eyes closed. Briony said: "As soon as she was in the correct position, her breathing became markedly laboured and her neck really ached and hurt. As the correction progressed, these symptoms eased until there was no sign of them at all - then the correction was completed. Her breathing by this time was relaxed and deep." When she went home, the client told her husband about the work that had been done, and he said that the position established through muscle testing was exactly how the paramedics found her. After the correction her neck stopped hurting in the mornings, and the client felt more relaxed in general.

"The improvement over night was astonishing."

One day I went to my tai chi class, and I slipped: both my feet went up in the air in front of me, and I landed on my right wrist. I ended up with a displaced Colles' fracture [a break in the radius bone just above the wrist]. I depend on my right hand – I'm a cartoonist and illustrator. I was put into theatre to twist it back, and then it was in plaster for about four weeks. When the plaster came off, the damn hand wouldn't work. It was mottled, swollen, and painful, and my palm was sweaty. Noticeable hair was

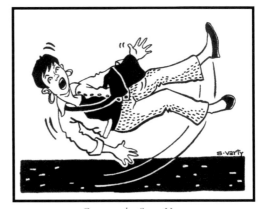

Cartoon by Suzy Varty

growing on the back of my hand. I couldn't do the exercise the physio gave me – thumb to base of little finger – nowhere near. At the fracture clinic they said they thought I had RSD – reflex sympathetic dystrophy – an auto-immune response. Even five months after the accident there wasn't a lot of difference.

I went to see Christine, because I thought she could sort out some vitamins to help the healing process. Christine asked if I'd got over the trauma, and I said that I still felt shocked by it – I'd never broken anything before. Christine tested and found that I needed a body position memory – I re-enacted the position I ended up in. I realised that I felt angry - I had just come back from the States and pushed myself to go to tai chi even though I didn't really want to, and then this happened. Next day when I got up it was 95% better – the improvement over night was astonishing. It's made a big difference. Now I can use it without any problem. It's fine – except if it's damp I can feel the break and it gets a bit stiff, so I'm going to see if Christine can improve that.

Client *Suzy Varty* and Practitioner *Christine Fowler*

Operations

Health kinesiology treatment can mean that a planned operation becomes unnecessary, or, if the operation is still needed, HK can often be used to help counteract some of the stress and discomfort of surgery.

> A client with a chronic lung condition needed an operation for an unrelated problem. She was very anxious about this, and extra precautions were being taken with the anaesthetic because of her lung problems. We did HK to help her cope with her fears before the operation. I also worked out a programme of homeopathic remedies to be taken before and after the operation. The outcome was that she coped very well with the operation and made a good recovery.

Scars

HK practitioners can help incision wounds to heal more quickly. If the operation was some time ago, scar corrections are likely to be necessary, but in the immediate aftermath of an operation spin corrections (see page 65) and electromagnetic field corrections (see page 64) will often help the body to heal quickly with the minimum discomfort.

> Denise Kilonsky helped her father after his triple heart bypass surgery, when he was experiencing a great deal of pain from the incisions in his chest and leg. About a week after the surgery his incisions became very painful. They burned, itched and ached deep in his chest. An electromagnetic field correction was needed using two tiny magnets: one at the top of his chest incision and one at the bottom. He said: "After the HK treatment the pain decreased and was completely gone within two days."

> A spin correction was also needed on the incision in the crease of his leg. Denise's father said: "I was experiencing pain from both the hardening incision scab, and from the muscles and nerves that had been cut to remove the vein. The scab pain went away instantly, but the pain of the cut muscles and nerves took longer to clear."

Scars often bother people for cosmetic reasons, or because they cause discomfort, but they may have a far deeper significance for the energy system. Scar corrections can make a dramatic difference, because scars can interfere with the smooth flow of energy in the meridians.

If a scar crosses a meridian, it can disturb the flow of energy in that meridian. The bigger the scar, the more likely this is to happen, but even small scars can have a big impact if their position is across a meridian, particularly if an acupuncture point is involved. Disturbing the meridian energy flow can lead to problems in the physical body. When I published an article on this topic, many people wrote to me to say that they had not felt right since having an operation, but had felt unable to say anything to anyone. The letters often expressed relief that the article suggested a reason for this and could validate their experience.

If a scar is a problem on an energy level, it will often not have healed well, appearing raised or discoloured, for example. There is often altered sensation at or around the site - numbness, coldness or a feeling that the area does not 'belong' to the body.

HK has a specific procedure for healing scars. It involves the person touching the scar in a particular way with one or more fingers (established using muscle testing), while the energy system is rebalanced. Many people experience redness, itching, discomfort and even pain in the area of the scar in the two or three days following this type of work. Sometimes small spots full of pus appear along the scar line. Clients often say that it feels as though the body is completing the healing that should have been done at the time of the operation or accident. This can be the case even with scars that are many years old.

Subsequently there is often a feeling that the scarred area has been reintegrated into the whole body. Any numbness or coldness will usually disappear, regardless of how old the scar is. Often there are also improvements in the appearance of the scar; for example, it may become less prominent, and the colour may become more like that of the surrounding skin.

"As ... qualified nurses ... we would not have believed that any physical signs of healing would start to emerge so quickly."

While I was studying HK, I volunteered for a scar correction demonstration done on the first day of a four-day workshop. I was particularly bothered by my scar, which happened whilst serving with the Royal Navy during the Falklands war. Despite the duration of time that had elapsed since the surgery, the scar was still deep pink and very taut. It was also devoid of any sensation, as was the whole area for five centimetres below the scar line.

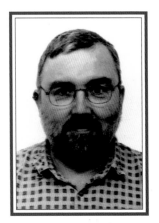

The scar itself was twenty centimetres long running from my midline down along the ribcage ending on my right side and was at least one centimetre wide over the whole length. Jane tested that there were three corrections to do in all, but that it was OK for her to complete only the first one as a demonstration. Whilst Jane and some of the other students held points, I felt very relaxed but was not aware of any physical sensations in or around the scar. However, within around thirty minutes of the correction I felt a sensation of warmth at the site of the scar and the whole area of skin surrounding it had become flushed! As my wife and I are both qualified nurses, trained to be objective and scientific, we would not have believed that any physical signs of healing would start to emerge so quickly.

Amazingly, throughout the day the colour of that part of the scar that had been 'corrected' had begun to fade and it seemed that each time another student wanted to look at the scar it was quite apparent that changes were taking place. I began to feel quite distracted around lunchtime, finding it hard to concentrate on anything at all and I was very glad when the day was over and my wife (also a HK student) and I could go to our hotel away from everyone. During the evening, I was restless and could not settle to read or watch TV. My wife tested to see if the other two corrections needed to be done, but they were to be done four days later when we would be back at home. For the rest of the night I was restless and did not sleep well. By the next morning I felt more unfocussed - but the scar itself continued to change its appearance and the actual stitch marks were very evident, little white dots either side of the scar!

I was completely unable to concentrate during the class that morning. By lunchtime I had become aware that the reason I was feeling so restless was that memories and feelings attached to the scar and events during my time in the Falklands were surfacing. I became increasingly distressed and felt that I could not continue with the workshop - I wanted to run and hide. Fortunately, my wife would not let me and asked Jane to help me in dealing with these feelings as by this time I was in tears. Jane did the necessary work using cosbats, and by the time the afternoon session began I was feeling much more like my usual self. I hadn't realised how powerful the scar correction would be, but I know that your energy system only gives you work that you can deal with safely.

The appearance of the scar continued to change over the next two days, sometimes pink, sometimes white, I had a very faint pink rash over the skin at one point and the scar itself became less taut. On day three I had some sensation in my skin around the scar for the first time in sixteen years!

My wife did the remaining corrections once we were home and we had been so impressed by the occurrences during the workshop that we bought a Polaroid camera in order to photograph further changes! I did not experience any further psychological distress during or after these corrections, but the scar turned deep pink again for twenty-four hours and then began to fade. We checked the scar everyday and the appearance altered everyday in some way. Within two weeks I regained full sensation around the scar. Three months on, eight centimetres of the scar from the midline have completely faded making it difficult to see at all, the width reduced to just four millimetres. The remaining twelve centimetres continue to fade and I am delighted that the scar I have today bears no resemblance at all to the one I wanted correcting.

Before beginning to study HK we would never have believed this to be possible despite (or because of) all our years of medical/nursing experience. We both have total faith in HK and feel that anything is possible within this truly holistic process and we look forward to the time when HK is being practised in hospitals and GP surgeries. It is something that should be accessible to all.

Practitioner *Bob Williams*

Scar work can even lead to more superficial scars disappearing altogether. While treating a client for respiratory problems, I did some energy work on a scar caused by a scratch from the family's cat. The scar was fairly superficial but had been there for about two months. Although it was not the cause of the client's problems, it was interfering with the flow of energy through the lung meridian and hampering the body's attempts to rebalance itself. By the time my client reached home, about an hour after the energy work on the scar had been completed, the scar had completely disappeared.

Scar corrections can produce some very dramatic results.

A twenty-nine-year-old woman came to see me about a spectacular skin rash. It had started with a few spots on her chest and two days later spots had developed all over her body. Eventually the spots had dried and crusty scabs had formed, leaving her skin looking as though she had a bad case of psoriasis. Her GP and the skin specialist were mystified and finally attributed the problem to a course of sunbed treatments she had just completed. When I take a case history, I always ask about operations and accidents. The client told me that a mole had been removed from the inside of her right thigh ten days before the skin problem started. The scar was very small and neat, but it ran directly across the liver meridian. Through muscle testing I established that the scar was disturbing her liver meridian energy and was causing her physical liver to function less well. This meant that metabolic by-products normally broken down by the liver were instead being excreted through the skin leading to the severe skin rash. I used corrections to rebalance the energy around the scar and to support her liver, and the rash disappeared very quickly.

Major scars can have a profound and permanent effect on a person's life unless the energy imbalances they create are put right.

My eldest son, Jon, provides a wonderful example of the benefits that can be achieved when energy work is done on scars. Jon was born with an exomphalos, which means that the midline of the body does not join and sometimes, as in his case, some of the internal organs are outside the body. At that time, many children died from this condition, and Jon needed immediate major surgery. This left him with one very large scar (over seven inches long) and other subsidiary scarring on his torso. There are several meridians running up and down the torso: the central meridian, the liver meridian, the kidney meridian, the spleen meridian and the stomach meridian. Jon had a very small appetite and preferred to eat little and often rather than having a normal meal. I had difficulty finding trousers that were comfortable for him to wear, because the waistbands tended to rub the scar. He was also severely dyslexic.

I first used health kinesiology on Jon when he was eight years old, at the time I was first introduced to the system. The main scar from his first operation when he was eight hours old was still red and raised with a lot of keloidal tissue. After working on this scar Jon's dyslexia improved. The redness of the scar disappeared, and much of the keloidal tissue was reabsorbed. Jon also started to eat more. When I discussed this with him, he told me that he used to feel that his stomach would burst open if he ate a lot. (He had thought this was normal, because it had always been the case for him.) The energy work on his scar changed all that. It also improved the energy flow through the torso meridians in general and through the central meridian in particular. Interestingly, the central meridian is involved with the brain, so this may be the reason for that first dramatic improvement in his dyslexia (see the Introduction). There is still a distinctive scar on his torso, but it no longer causes him any discomfort.

Scars do not only affect the physical body, they can also have profound effects on a person's sense of emotional well-being, because meridian imbalances may have a psychological effect.

A woman whose problems included obsessiveness, allowing small things to overwhelm her, and constantly checking things consulted me. She lacked self-confidence and often apologized repeatedly even when she knew she was not responsible. Our first appointment was very short, and we only had time to do a little piece of work, involving rebalancing the energy of a scar on her right foot (the result of a bunion operation). This scar was in the area of the spleen meridian. According to *Zen Shiatsu* by S Masunago and W Ohashi imbalances associated with this meridian include over-concern for details, restlessness associated with anxiety, and a tendency to over eat. When the client came for her next appointment a month later, she told me that she was not checking things so much, and that both her husband and her mother had noticed the change in her. With further HK work she became progressively calmer, less obsessive and more self-confident. She also lost twenty eight pounds in weight.

I believe that in an ideal world the best of conventional medical treatment would be supported by health kinesiology to minimize drug reactions and pre- and post- operational stress, to stimulate healing and to repair scarring.

12: Homework: Helping People To Help Themselves

Sometimes the energy work completed during the appointments is all that is needed to restore health, but sometimes the client has to do something themselves after the session. This 'homework' is found through muscle testing and usually comes under the energy toning category (see page 60) or adjunctive factors (see page 60).

Homework comes in many different forms. For example, clients sometimes have to take something or wear something; an exercise or rest programme worked out during the session might need to be carried out in the succeeding days or weeks. The precise form of the homework is determined through muscle testing.

Diet And Nutritional Supplements

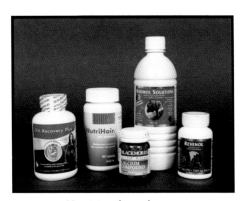

Nutritional supplements

Diet and nutrition are categorized under adjunctive factors and may come up during a session as a result of muscle testing. Sometimes clients will specifically ask practitioners for advice on how to improve their diet or what supplements to take. Nutrition and diet can come up during a session as a result of verbal questioning and muscle testing. In either case what dietary changes and exactly which supple-ments and what dosage are established using muscle testing. The practitioner's nutritional knowledge may suggest suitable supplements or a diet regime, but this is always confirmed by muscle testing. A client may need to eat a particular food, drink more water, or eat at a different time of day in order to achieve their goal. Alternatively, they may need to stop doing something – stop eating a particular food for a while or stop taking a supplement.

Energy corrections had helped a client with severe facial eczema to make some progress. Then we had one session where muscle testing showed that only one adjunctive factor was required: the client needed to take two teaspoons of walnut oil each day. Within a very short time the eczema on her face had completely cleared.

Another client, whose psoriasis was responding well to HK treatment, phoned to say she was much worse again. I arranged to see her, and muscle testing quickly made it clear that she had started to do something new and that had caused the problem. She volunteered that she had started to take cod liver oil for her arthritis. Testing showed that it was indeed this had caused her psoriasis to flare up again. This problem was quickly solved: she stopped taking the cod liver oil, and we booked her an appointment to start working on her arthritis.

Psoriasis And Arthritis

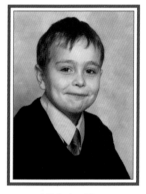

Nicholas Hyett

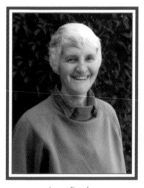

Ann Parker

Nicholas Hyett was eight when he came to see me. He had psoriasis, and it was so bad that his back often bled at night. He came for six sessions during the year, and from one session to the next there was steady improvement in his skin condition. His father had left the family when Nicholas was eighteen months old. The HK work was able to deal very gently with his emotional pain. He had to give up the fizzy drinks, start drinking six glasses of water a day, and change his diet. His mother was so impressed with the results that she came as a client herself to deal with her asthma.

I also helped another client, Paul, with his psoriasis. He had had psoriasis for thirty years and was now covered with it, but initially he consulted me about his severe arthritis. Paul had been unable to work as a carpenter for several months due to it. By the third visit he was back at work as his hands had healed. Then he was keen to see if health kinesiology could help him sort out his psoriasis. Muscle testing showed he needed to make changes in his diet. He came every three to four months for a further two years and, as we worked on underlying emotional problems, the skin gradually improved. When I last saw him, his skin was clear and had been for about three years.

Clients *Nicholas Hyett* and *"Paul"*, and Practitioner *Ann Parker*

Rest

HK makes a clear distinction between rest and relaxation. Relaxation includes activities such as watching television, going for a gentle walk, gardening at a leisurely pace, and so on. Rest is an absence of activity of any kind. So, for example, listening to music is not rest, but it is relaxation (if the music is pleasurable). Rest supports the physical body, and so is classified as an adjunctive factor.

Most people do not rest enough. When the energy system asks for rest, many clients will say that they do not have time. However, experience shows that if people rest as they should, they often need much less sleep. In many cases fifteen minutes rest a day can reduce the need for sleep by as much as an hour, so taking the right amount of rest could actually mean having more time to do things, rather than less. The optimum rest schedule is established through muscle testing.

Exercise

Studies have shown that the health benefits of exercise include improved cardiovascular fitness, reduced risk of osteoporosis and pre-menopausal breast cancer, better weight control and an enhanced self-image.

Health kinesiology can determine the right exercise programme for each individual. As with most things, there is no single ideal routine that suits everyone. Different people need different mixes of aerobic exercise, strength training and flexibility exercises.

As well as working with people who want to use exercise to improve their overall health, HK can also help the competitive athlete or sports person to tailor their training schedule so that they maximize their performance goals without risking injury or a compromised immune system.

> Practitioner Judy Gavan's son, Ben, injured his wrist during a weight training session. His training schedule had consisted of lifting weights for one hour on alternate days, and on the other days completing one hour of press-ups. With input from Ben on all the different possibilities, Judy worked out a new schedule. This involved reducing the weight-lifting sessions to forty minutes twice a week, reducing each weight by ten pounds, and doing only twenty minute sessions of press-ups twice a week. Muscle testing also revealed that to balance the stamina-building exercises, Ben needed some aerobic exercise: an hour of swimming twice a week was included in the programme. Ben's wrist was fully healed in two weeks, and he decided to keep to the new exercise programme, as it felt far more enjoyable and more beneficial to his general health and well-being than the previous regime.

> One young client had been having physiotherapy every week for over a year. One of her legs was shorter than the other, probably due to a misaligned pelvis. Her energy system asked for an exercise programme, so we used muscle testing to work out the correct activity specifically for her. She had to spend fifteen minutes each day doing particular exercises, and within one week her legs had become the same length.

Wearing Magnets

As well as using magnets for correction procedures such as electric current corrections (see page 62), clients may need to wear one or more magnets for a while (adjunctive factors). The south-seeking pole of a magnet sedates and calms, and the north-seeking pole stimulates - this effect can be used to enhance healing. If body processes are sluggish, causing for example swelling or pus formation, putting the north-seeking pole of a magnet over the affected area will speed up body processes and encourage healing. If there is too much activity, such as pain and cramping, a north-seeking magnet will have a calming effect. Of course, the health kinesiologist does not decide which pole to use intellectually but muscle tests carefully. Sometimes even in cases of over activity the north-seeking pole is used. In these cases the energy system is using the magnet to enhance an existing process and bring it to a speedy resolution. I have used magnets with great success to help pain, leg ulcers and one case of repetitive strain injury.

> Practitioner Amanda Pollard helped her aunt, Ellie Carter, who had been suffering from a pain in her shoulder for over a year. Amanda tested that her aunt needed to wear four small disc magnets on the painful shoulder for fifteen days. On the fourteenth night, while she was in bed, her shoulder made a loud noise, and it immediately felt better. It has been fine ever since.

Flower Remedies And Homepathic Remedies

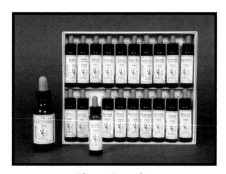
Flower Remedies

Flower remedies and homeopathic remedies sometimes form part of an SET procedure (see page 111), but HK practitioners also use them in the traditional way as a remedy to be taken. This may be only once, but sometimes on a daily basis for several weeks or months.

The remedy is identified through muscle testing, and although it may make sense in terms of its traditional use, it sometimes makes no obvious sense at all.

On one occasion my youngest son, Tom, had a bad cough and testing showed that he needed a homeopathic remedy. I carefully tested my box of homeopathic remedies without looking at the labels on the bottles and found that he needed 'symphytum'. I looked this up in one of my homeopathy books and discovered that symphytum was the Latin name for comfrey or knitbone. As the traditional name suggests, this is usually a remedy for broken bones. It is also used in the treatment of ulcers, head pains and injuries to the eye, but no chest or respiratory symptoms were listed for it. This happened many years ago, before I had the confidence in HK that I have now, so I decided not to give Tom the remedy. By the next day his cough was much worse, so again I muscle tested to find out what would help him. The answer was still a homeopathic remedy, so again I tested the bottles without looking at the labels. Again symphytum came up. This time I gave Tom the remedy and within a couple of hours his cough had gone completely.

Life Transformers

Life transformers are gemstones (such as rose quartz, aventurine and sodalite) that have been energetically modified and enhanced so that they permanently carry a particular psychological or energy-protective quality. There are many different ones, including those for *confidence, overcoming fears, protection from other people's energies, protection from electromagnetic pollution* and *success*. Dr Jimmy Scott, the developer of HK, created them so that people who were not able to consult a health kinesiologist could wear one and still enjoy some of the benefits, although in a more limited way. Life transformers are still used in this way, but they are also used to enhance and reinforce the energy corrections done by the practitioner.

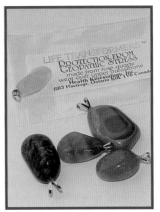

Life Transformers

Practitioner Pan Wade identified a life transformer for her granddaughter Grace. Pan says: "She was objectionable from the age of ten months; she was jealous of her brother and later on of her younger sister; she sulked endlessly and had temper tantrums." Pan tested that her granddaughter would benefit from the life transformer *coping with jealousy*. Grace was very suspicious of the stone and refused to wear it, but she slept with it under her pillow. It took some time, but eventually Grace changed significantly. In Pan's words: "She became such a sweetie to have around." Both Pan and Grace's mother are convinced that the transformation of Grace is, at least partly, due to the life transformer.

Life transformers can even be helpful for animals.

A budgerigar became ill every time its owner went away. The owner became very distressed and was reluctant to leave the budgie. Once the Life Transformer *overcoming depression* was hung in the bird's cage there were no further problems, and the owner was able to enjoy her holidays, knowing that her pet would be well on her return.

Life transformers can also be used in energy corrections during a consultation. This can be an effective way of rapidly correcting a lot of psychological stresses. Muscle testing shows which life transformers to use, and where on the body to position them. Acupuncture points are held or cosmic batteries are used to complete the correction.

Affirmations

An affirmation is a statement about what the client wants to achieve, but said as though it is true now. It has to be said with as much conviction as possible. Affirmations are part of energy toning. Like all other procedures in HK, they are tailor-made for each individual client. Muscle testing is used to establish the exact wording, the number of repetitions and all other details, such as if the affirmation has to be said out loud in a particular place or in front of a mirror.

Sometimes the affirmation is very precise and clear, e.g. *I am independent and free*, but sometimes it is more ambiguous, such as *Life begins*. One client had to say out loud, several times each day: *God protects me*. Whatever the affirmation chosen by the energy system it always seems to be perfect for the person and their needs.

A woman who was seven months pregnant consulted an HK practitioner in New York. At the end of the session an affirmation came up as her homework. The statement was: *Natural childbirth is attainable*. The client did not believe that a vaginal birth would be possible, as she had been told that the child was very large, and she should prepare herself for a caesarean section. For the rest of her pregnancy the client diligently repeated the affirmation each day. Finally a beautiful 10 lbs. 15 oz baby girl was born vaginally after a relatively quick labour.

A client, who as a child had been abused by her mother, consulted practitioner Hattie Warner. Her mother would tread on her daughter's toes, hit her with a wooden spoon, lock her in a cupboard under the stairs, and denigrate her in front of her younger brother. Her father did nothing. The client had tried to commit suicide in her teens and would now panic when she was left in a room on her own. Hattie completed a phobia correction and then an affirmation came up: *I cherish my beautiful inner child*. The work and the affirmation have transformed the client's life, and she is now much more confident and happy. Her relationships with her parents and her brother have also improved.

Visualizations

Visualizations are also part of energy toning and involve the client imagining something that they want to achieve as though it is true now. Again, all the details of the item are established through muscle testing.

Practitioner Shahzadi Thomas was consulted by a woman whose marriage had ended, and who was having to leave the marital home. She was very sad about this, and afraid she would never find another home she liked as much. Muscle testing revealed that she needed a visualization of a new home, created from the most important features of her existing home, with the addition of others to accommodate her new future. Testing found that she needed to visualize this every morning for the next ten days. Within two weeks she had details of lots of houses, most of which contained about eighty per cent of the requirements from the visualization. Very shortly afterwards she found a house, which fulfilled ninety five per cent of her needs and wants for a home. She bought the house and now lives there very happily.

Meridian Tracing

Some clients get a programme of exercises to tone the physical body, and others get a programme of exercises to tone their energy system. In meridian tracing the acupuncture meridians are traced lightly with the fingers either on the body or just off the body. Sometimes all the meridians need to be traced and sometimes the client has to trace only one. The frequency and duration are established through muscle testing. This 'homework' is relatively quick to do, and people often feel lighter and more awake afterwards, as well as seeing more long-term benefits.

> Katheline Bouchery of Belgium helped a long-standing client, Françoise Brison, after a fall in the garden. Her left wrist was swollen and she had a big bruise on her left shin. Katheline found that Françoise needed to complete the meridian tracing exercises. Then Katheline did two spin corrections on her. By the next day the swelling in her wrist had gone down and the bruise was less tender.

HK Energy Toning Movements

Many different branches of kinesiology use meridian tracing, but energy toning movements are specific to HK, and were devised by Jimmy Scott. They are designed to strengthen and tone the meridians, and normally each movement is completed about seven times. As with meridian tracing, it may be that only one or two toning movements are necessary. One small client with a runny nose had to do the movement related to the lung meridian twice each day. Fortunately this particular movement is relatively easy to do and she was very happy to copy her mother.

> Reti Winward only needed to see a client once for insomnia. The client had been unable to sleep properly for many months. It took her hours to get to sleep and then she would wake a couple of hours later and be unable to go back to sleep again. The issue title was: *I Need To Relax*. The only corrections needed were tissue energy blocks. These were followed by some energy toning movements. That evening she fell asleep while watching television and, having transferred to her bed, slept right through till the morning. After that she fell asleep easily every night and, when Reti next saw her about a year later, she was still sleeping well.

Electromagnetic Pollution And Degaussing

We live in a world in which electromagnetic pollution is unavoidable. The phenomenal growth in home computers, personal stereo players, mobile phones and battery-operated watches has contributed to this problem. Even those who do not have any of this modern equipment are still exposed to the radio and television waves that travel through the air. Televisions and radios simply receive and change the signals that are present in the air, whether or not the equipment is being used.

Some people seem relatively immune to this major change in our environment, but others know to their cost how sensitive they are to it. They pay the price every day in the form of headaches, difficulty concentrating, and so on. It is possible to be severely affected by electromagnetic pollution but unaware that this is the source of the symptoms.

Those who are very sensitive to electromagnetic pollution often have a tendency to receive static electric shocks. They may find it extremely difficult to switch off the television, even when what the programme is of no interest, and may be 'addicted' to video games.

HK can help a person to become less sensitive to electromagnetic pollution. The client with chronic fatigue syndrome described on page 98 came to see me to get her allergies fixed, but the primary work focused on making her less sensitive to electromagnetic pollution. When we did this, her allergies completely disappeared. This happened very quickly after the first session, but it can take some people a long time to become robust in the face of this new and insidious form of pollution. For those people a temporary solution is provided by eliminating residual electromagnetic fields in the body, or 'degaussing'.

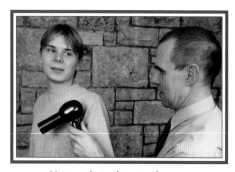

Using a hair drier to degausse

Degaussing involves a simple but seemingly odd procedure where a small electric motor is passed briefly over the whole of the body. For most people a hairdryer provides a suitable motor. This usually needs to be done on a regular basis, often once a week. It takes only a few minutes and people often report feeling more 'awake' when they start doing it regularly. Problems with static electric shocks seem to disappear and people often become much less 'addicted' to television and video games.

Testing showed that degaussing was appropriate for some friends who were complaining that they found it impossible to switch off the television. The whole family would sit staring at the screen like zombies. Initially they obviously thought degaussing was a totally improbable solution, but decided that for the sake of our friendship they would humour me. They were amazed at the difference it made the first time. Subsequently, they arranged family degaussing sessions whenever they started to find it difficult to switch off the television.

The mother of a young client told me she had started suffering from headaches. She was working part-time in front of a computer, and each day she would return home with a headache. I suggested she tried degaussing with a hairdryer. When her son came for his next appointment six weeks later, she told me that she had not had a single headache since she had been degaussing regularly.

There are many different possibilities for things that people can do to help themselves. Because the HK practitioner uses muscle testing, the precise programme that the individual needs can be worked out accurately. Clients are much more likely to do homework that is worked out in this way: it is tailored to them and their needs, and results are likely to be evident more quickly than if they just did something that in general works for people with similar problems.

> ## "I was a little sceptical, but ... within two days my back had eased considerably"
>
> I have worked in the building trade for most of my life. I am now forty one and have had various degrees of back trouble – some minor and some more serious where I have had to have short periods of time off work. I have never visited a doctor because all they seem to prescribe is painkillers, which I see as masking the pain and not curing the problem.
>
> I was doing some particularly heavy work when my back went again. I managed to keep working for a couple of days but I found if I stayed in one position for too long I "seized up". This made sitting down, sleeping and particularly getting out of bed in the morning a long and painful experience.
>
> I decided to seek help. This is when I visited Sandra Shackleton. The treatment I had was HK, which was non-intrusive, painless and lasted about forty five minutes. I was a little sceptical, but after the treatment I went home and rested. Within two days my back had eased considerably and within three days I was working again, and within a week I was able to sit, sleep and get out of bed with no pain at all.
>
> At the time of writing (ten months later) I have had no trouble at all with my back despite doing some very heavy work and participating in sport.
>
> Client *Brian Jennings* and Practitioner *Sandra Shackleton*

13: The Future

When I first became a kinesiologist no one seemed to have heard of it. When asked what I did, I would say: "I'm a kinesiologist, but you won't know what that is, so I'll explain." After doing this for about four years, someone replied: "But I do know what that is." I did not believe them, and said: "No, you must be thinking of something else." It turned out that this person **did** know about kinesiology, so I started to alter what I said.

Over the succeeding years more and more people have known what a kinesiologist is. Now replies include: "Oh yes, I saw something about that on the TV", or "My chiropractor does that", or even "My sister is going to see one."

Kinesiology is becoming recognized as a fascinating and powerful therapy, but there is still some way to go.

I have many dreams for the future of health kinesiology:

- The National Health Service will include regular BBEI check-ups for babies from conception to two months of age.

- Doctors will check through muscle testing for adverse reactions to drugs before prescribing.

- Surgeons will test for the least damaging place to cut before performing operations, and kinesiologists will be available to help the body heal as quickly as possible.

- Dentists will check before fitting a brace that it will not cause electric current problems for the patient. If a problem exists, they will know how to correct it.

- People who easily become addicted to television, computers and video games will regularly degauss themselves so that they can develop wider interests.

- Athletes will tap their sports performance potential, not with illicit drugs, but by using safe and effective kinesiology techniques.

- Parents, step-parents and carers of very young children will be offered a simple test to check if they are stressed by the sound of a baby crying. If they are, simple HK procedures will be used to correct the problem.

- Kinesiologists will work alongside veterinarians to offer simple safe effective help to animals.

- Doctors in general practice will be aware of kinesiology and know when it is appropriate to refer patients for this therapy.

- Teachers will recognize that some children are not lazy or stupid – they need the help that a kinesiologist can offer.

- People will not need to follow complicated diets in order to avoid allergy problems, but that they will consult a kinesiologist and have the problem solved.

- Anyone who is overweight will be checked to see if the body is miscategorizing body chemicals, and simple HK procedures will be used to solve the problem and avoid the misery of dieting, poor health and low self-esteem that excess weight brings for so many people.

- When people want to help themselves, by following an exercise or diet plan for example, they will consult a kinesiologist to find out what is the very best programme for them to follow.

- There will be a kinesiology practitioner in every town, and kinesiology will be a household name, a therapy of first choice.

How To Become A Health Kinesiology Practitioner

It is not necessary to be medically qualified to become a health kinesiology practitioner, or even to have any formal academic qualifications. However, health kinesiology is a logical, rigorous system demanding clear and precise thinking. The training requires a high level of commitment and application, but enables students to build their knowledge and skills in progressive steps.

The basic system is taught in five stages, with a four-day course for each. These courses are usually spaced about two to three months apart, but students can work at their own pace, taking much longer if more convenient. All the teachers work to the same syllabus, using the same manuals (in translation if necessary). Students can take different courses with different teachers, if they wish, but the courses must be taken in a particular order. Students must also complete case studies and provide evidence of extensive home study. The teacher regularly monitors students' progress through the stages, and there is a final assessment day. Most practitioners take one and a half to two years to become qualified, although some take longer, and Nancy Booth (see page 148) took less time.

The UK training programme is accredited by the Open College Network, which provides an independent moderator. The training is also approved by the Kinesiology Federation, the main professional body in Britain for kinesiologists, as providing suitable professional training in kinesiology. Practitioners in the UK also have to complete additional courses in anatomy and physiology, practice management, counselling and nutrition to be accredited by the Kinesiology Federation. The KF is affiliated to the British Complementary Medicine Association (BCMA), which represents many different branches of complementary therapy.

The basic system is made up of the following five stages, which are studied in this order.

Stage 1

Initial balancing of the acupuncture energy system, psychological corrections, allergy and tolerance testing and correction (the tapping technique), basic treatment protocols.

Stage 2

Further training in allergy and tolerance work, procedures for detoxifying the body (the SET technique), electric current corrections, electromagnetic field corrections, spin corrections, using magnets as an adjunctive, self-testing.

"HK is good fun to do and you can help yourself with it too."

My name is Alice Morgan, my Mum, Sue, is a health kinesiologist. My Mum works on me because I have had catarrh since I was a baby and it blocks up my ears and nose and makes me cough. When she does HK work on me it helps me to feel much better and I can hear properly.

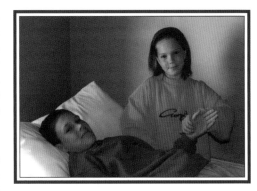

Mum has a room in the house where she works with her clients. I am so proud of her when she helps people get better, that I wanted to do it too. So, I made part of my bedroom into an HK corner. I practiced on my dolls and I even had a file to keep all my work in. I used to copy how Mum made her notes.

After that Mum taught me how to do a balancing tap and energy toning movements. I sometimes balance my friends in the playground at school. They think it's fun too.

My mum showed me how to fight my catarrh using a hairdryer back to front so that the air blows away from me and going all around my body, isn't that clever? Oh and by the way it makes me feel better in the morning, then I can start my day without being wheezy. I have to be careful not to catch my hair in the hairdryer though!

I really like having a Mum who's a health kinesiologist because she helps me, my brothers and my Dad stay well and healthy. HK is good fun to do and you can help yourself with it too.

Alice Morgan Age 9

Stage 3

Powerful psychological corrections (including the being/not being structure and the gerund structure) scars and pain corrections, some energy flow balancing corrections, issue analysis and facet analysis.

Stage 4

More psychological corrections, working with life transformers, more energy flow balancing corrections, affirmations, energy toning movements, etc.

Stage 5

Further psychological techniques (including the linked opposite, imperative and phobia corrections), chakra rebalancing procedures, more energy flow balancing corrections, designing exercise programmes, etc.

Advanced Courses

There are currently five advanced courses (stages 6-10). In some countries Stage 6, which includes more advanced techniques, is also included in the initial training, although this is not the case in the UK. Most practitioners are keen to learn more and are eager to attend the advanced workshops in order to further their skills.

The precise detail of the training programme may be different in some other countries.

"I just knew this was IT for me."

I read an article on health kinesiology by Jane Alexander – a *Daily Mail* journalist. I just knew this was IT for me. To be able to speak to a body – via muscle testing – for me was the ultimate! The article was very timely. At work British Gas were looking for people to take voluntary redundancy – part of the package being a retraining scheme. To cut a long story short, I left British Gas. They paid for my training in health kinesiology.

The teacher was wonderful and all our group bonded together – we became close friends, because we experienced so much together. I had to study hard, but the courses were well organised. I enjoyed discovering about myself through HK. By learning about myself it put me in a better position to help other people. I practiced mainly on friends, and they were very encouraging because what came up was very meaningful for them.

I applied for and received a local enterprise grant to help start up my business. I was up and running as an HK therapist within a year to the day of leaving work. After six years I am still enjoying my work and still very much in awe of the process.

Practitioner *Nancy C Booth*

Useful Addresses

Finding an HK practitioner and further information on HK training in the UK

Health Kinesiology UK
Sea View House, Long Rock, Penzance, TR20 8JF, England
Tel: 01736 719030; from outside the UK: +44 1736 719030
Fax: 01736 719040; from outside the UK: +44 1736 719040
Email: office@healthk.co.uk
Web site: www.healthk.co.uk

Finding an HK practitioner and further information on HK training elsewhere

Health Kinesiology International Headquarters
RR3 Hastings, Ontario, KOL 1YO, Canada
Tel: +1 705 696 3176
Fax: +1 705 696 3664
Email: hk@subtlenergy.com
Web site: www.subtlenergy.com

Jane Thurnell-Read's personal web site: www.lifeworkpotential.com

This web site includes information of interest both to the general public and kinesiology practitioners and students.

The Kinesiology Federation

The KF is the professional association for practitioners of different branches of kinesiology in Britain.

The Kinesiology Federation
PO Box 17153, Edinburgh, EH11 3WQ
Tel/Fax: 08700 113545
Email: kfadmin@kinesiologyfederation.org
Web site: www.kinesiologyfederation.org

Reading

By The Author

Geopathic Stress: How Earth Energies Affect Our Lives
Element Books Ltd., 1999, ISBN 1852306963
Unfortunately this book is currently out of print, because the publisher, Element Books, went out of business. Another publisher plans to reprint it.

This book is also available in other languages:

Les harmonies magnétiques	ISBN 2841144097
Geopatogénny Stres	ISBN 8085752530
Wie Erdstrahlen unser Leben beeinflussen	ISBN 3442139597
Stresul Teluric	ISBN 973601598X
Geopatogenni Zóny Kolem Nás	ISBN 8085809532
Le Energie Negative Della Terra	ISBN 8834410076

Other Kinesiology Books

Energy Medicine ISBN 0749919280	Donna Eden with David Feinstein
Instant Emotional Healing ISBN 0712606874	George Pratt
Kinesiology ISBN 072253454X	Maggie La Tourelle
Life Energy and The Emotions ISBN 1870845269	John Diamond
A Revolutionary Way of Thinking ISBN 0855722827	Dr Charles Krebs
Your Body Can Talk ISBN 0934252688	Susan L Levy

A comprehensive range of books on kinesiology and related subjects is for sale from:

Booklist, 78 Castlewood Drive, Eltham, London SE9 1NG
Tel/Fax: 020 8856 7717; Email: 1booklist@lineone.net

Glossary

Acupuncture meridian

See *meridian*.

Acupuncture points

Points on the *meridians* where energy may be effectively regulated. See also *holding acupuncture points*.

Acupuncture system

The system of *meridians* that supports life.

Acupuncture energy system

See *acupuncture system*.

Adjunctive factors

Activities that directly affect the physical body, and that clients will often do at home, e.g. taking a nutritional supplement, following an exercise programme, and so on. Compare *energy correction factors*, *energy toning factors*, *environmental factors* and *energy redirection factors*.

Affirmation

An *energy toning factor*. Positive statements that are repeated to a precise schedule. The schedule of repetitions and the exact wording of the affirmation is determined by muscle testing. Muscle testing is used to confirm that saying the affirmation is not stressful. If it is, then *energy work* is carried out first.

Allergen

The agent that sets off an allergic reaction.

Allergy

When exposure to any amount of a substance, however small, disturbs the person's energy flow, the person is said to have an allergy to that substance. The result is an altered reaction to that substance which may include physical and psychological symptoms. Medically allergy is defined as a hypersensitivity in which the body reacts with an exaggerated immune response without producing immunity. Compare with *tolerance*.

Allergy correction

Using the *allergy tap* or the *SET procedure* to rebalance the person's energy system while exposed to an *allergen*.

Allergy tap

A simple method for correcting allergies involving gently tapping specific acupuncture points while an allergen is placed on the client's body.

Anterior deltoid

A muscle in the shoulder that is often used as an *indicator muscle*.

Asking the body

See *asking verbal* questions.

Asking verbal questions

In HK this means the process of *asking verbal questions* while testing an *indicator muscle*. It is one of the most powerful ways of obtaining information from the body and determining how to help a person. The HK practitioner is trained to ask clear, logical, precise verbal questions and to interpret the results accurately. With the client's energy system balanced, the practitioner asks a verbal question either silently or out loud, and the client's *indicator muscle* is tested. A strong response indicates 'yes' and a weak response indicates 'no'. The meridian system must be in balance for the muscle to respond predictably.

Balancing around the navel

There are element test points for each meridian located around the navel. If one of these points is touched lightly and an indicator muscle tested at the same time, a weak response indicates over-energy in that *element*. If the point is touched firmly, a weakened indicator muscle shows under-energy in that element.

Balancing tap

See *thymus tap*.

Balancing the acupuncture system

See *initial balance*.

BBEIs

See *Body Brain Energy Integration*.

Being/Not Being correction

A type of *psychological correction*. It consists of at least two items. The first item is 'being X' and the next item is 'not being X'.

Body

This term is used to mean several different things depending on the context: a) the physical body itself, b) any of the various subtle energy bodies, and c) the complete individual including all physical and energy components.

Body Brain Energy Integration (BBEI)

A type of *energy correction* that is part of the sub-category of *energy control system correction*. These are simple, fundamental fears. They began before the client was two months of age. Although they look similar to *psychological corrections*, they are different in the way they affect the energy system.

Body position memory

A type of *energy correction* that is part of the sub-category of *energy flow balancing correction*. This is usually required as a result of severe stress or physical trauma. The result is that whenever a person is in a very specific body position then the acupuncture energy system becomes stressed. The body position memory correction removes the stress associated with the position.

Body priority

See *priority*.

Body sequence

See *overall body sequence*.

Brachioradialis

A muscle in the forearm that is often used as an *indicator muscle*.

Ch'i

The vital life force in the body taken in from the environment. It maintains all living cells. An imbalance of *yin* or *yang* can lead to a disruption in the smooth flow of Ch'i. The resulting imbalance may impair the functioning of physical cells.

Client specified issue

An *issue* to be addressed based on the concerns of the client and confirmed through muscle testing. Compare *HK tested issue*.

Cognitive sensory energy integration

A sub-category of *energy flow balancing corrections*, concerned with how the brain relates or integrates sensory information with cognitive processes.

Confirmation tests

The final steps of the initial balance. Once the practitioner thinks that the client is balanced, three confirmation tests are carried: yes/no, a magnet on an alternative muscle, and pinching an alternative muscle.

Conscious permission

A HK practitioner will not begin to work without conscious permission from the client. Normally, the client gives conscious permission by coming to the session. There is no hard and fast rule at what age children are capable of giving conscious permission. There may also be dilemmas as to whether someone who is mentally handicapped can give conscious permission. If it is felt this is not possible, an appropriate carer is asked to give conscious permission. See also *energy permission*.

Corrections

See *energy corrections*.

Cosbats

An abbreviation for *cosmic batteries*.

Cosmic batteries

A series of Belgian proprietary devices. Each cosmic battery is a glass tube containing an assortment of components, e.g. coils, coloured paper, symbols, homeopathic tablets. There are thirty four different ones. They provide *energy patterns* that can interact with an energy system so as to rebalance it. They can replace holding *acupuncture points* for *corrections*.

Coupled meridians

Meridians are coupled: a *yang* meridian with a *yin* meridian. Together they form an *element*.

Crystals

Can be used during a session or worn as *homework*. *Life transformers* are programmed crystals.

CSEI

See *cognitive sensory energy integration*.

Degaussing

A gauss is one unit of magnetic field strength. A hairdryer is used in HK temporarily to help desensitize a person to *electromagnetic fields*. (This does not mean that the person is magnetized and that they are being demagnetized.)

Diagnosis

Health kinesiology practitioners do not diagnose medical conditions. They look for energy imbalances that need correcting.

ECS

See *energy control system*.

EFB

See *energy flow balancing*.

Electric current

An electric current is produced when two dissimilar metals are in an electrolyte solution. Where metal in the body is in contact with a body fluid such as saliva, the resulting electric current can affect the body's own natural currents. The stress from this can be corrected permanently by electric current corrections.

Electromagnetic field

Whenever an electric current flows in a wire, a magnetic field is produced at right angles to the wire. Anything that plugs into an electrical supply, and most things that contain a battery, generate an electromagnetic field (EMF). The body itself has a weak electromagnetic field.

Electromagnetic field correction

A type of *energy correction*, which is part of the sub-category of *energy control system corrections*. These are needed where the body's own electromagnetic field is unbalanced in some way.

Element

In traditional Chinese philosophy everything is made up from five elements: wood, water, metal, earth and fire. Acupuncture meridians are organized into elements. HK uses seven elements, based on the traditional Chinese five-element theory, with the addition of the governing and central meridians (element 0 - air), and splitting the fire element into two parts (elements V and VI). Each element consists of a *yin meridian* and a *yang meridian*. (In modern science, 'element' has a different meaning from that used here.)

EMF correction

See *electromagnetic field correction*.

Energy

This term can be used to refer to physical body energy, or, more commonly in an HK context, to *subtle energy*.

Energy control system

This regulates and controls the flow of *energy* throughout the body, and so is one aspect of the *energy system*. It is electromagnetic in nature and can be disturbed by external electromagnetic fields and geopathic stress.

Energy correction

A procedure correcting imbalances in *energy patterns*. The practitioner identifies the *stressor* through muscle testing, triggers it in a controlled manner and removes the stress permanently by holding *acupuncture points* or using *cosmic batteries* to rebalance the *energy system*.

Energy correction factor

Energy work carried out by the practitioner, involving holding *acupuncture points* or placing *cosmic batteries* on the body. Compare *adjunctive factor, energy toning factor, environmental factors* and *energy redirection factor*.

Energy flow balancing

Types of *energy correction* directly concerned with improving the physical functioning of the body.

Energy meridian

See *meridian*.

Energy mismatch

When the energy system fails correctly to recognize the *energy pattern* of a substance.

Energy pattern

The characteristic array of energies associated with any given object, thought or substance. Everything has its own unique energy pattern and so is distinguishable from everything else. Similar things will have similar energy patterns, but there will still be some differences. It is the energy pattern of an object, thought or substance that interacts with an individual's own energy system.

Energy permission

Once the *initial balance* is complete, the practitioner asks for energy permission to work with the client. This is done by asking a verbal question and testing an *indicator muscle*.

Energy redirection factor

Used when the energy of the body needs to be encouraged to respond to new options that have become available, or in order to direct energy to some specific goal that may not be of the highest priority for the body. Compare *energy correction factors, energy toning factors, environmental factors* and *adjunctive factors*.

Energy toning movements

A series of movements, one for each *meridian*, used for energy toning. The effectiveness of these is not related to the physical movement involved, but rather to the effect on various components of the *energy system*.

Energy toning factor

Activities carried out by the client to tone the energy system rather than to affect the physical body. Compare *energy correction factor, energy redirection factor, environmental factor* and *adjunctive factor*.

Energy work

Work carried out to influence the *meridians* and the *subtle bodies*. Once this has happened the physical organs and systems may rebalance because of their dynamic relationship with the subtle bodies.

Environmental factor

The environmental factor covers reactions to environmental problems. This includes problems of environmental pollution and toxicity, and also geopathic stress problems. Compare *energy correction factor*, *energy redirection factor*, *energy toning factor* and *adjunctive factor*.

Etheric body

This is a copy of the physical body in energy form. It ensures that the foetus grows correctly and that physical repair and renewal are carried out appropriately.

Facet

An aspect of the issue being addressed. HK recognizes five facets, and uses them to help ensure that all aspects of the problem are covered. The five facets are: the cause facet, the effect facet, the process facet, the repair facet and the symptom facet.

Facet analysis

Analysing an *issue* in terms of the work that is necessary in each of the five *facets*.

Factor

A category of procedures within the HK system. See *HK menu*.

Flower remedies

These can be used during an appointment, or the client may have to take them at home. Flower remedies are prepared in a special way so that only the energetic qualities of the flower remain in the remedy. Taking specific ones can help the client to experience psychological and physical changes. The most famous (and the original) flower remedies are the ones produced by Dr Edward Bach. Also available are remedies made from the energy qualities of other things, such as trees, crystals and geographical locations (earth energies).

Gerund structure

A type of *energy correction* that is part of the sub-category *psychological corrections*. Each item begins with a gerund (a verb ending in 'ing').

Gizmo

An energy device worn to protect the individual from the effects of electromagnetic pollution. It is about the size of a large coin. Unfortunately these have been unavailable for some time. Practitioners who do have them may also use them for *spin* corrections.

Group

A related set of items for correction that have exactly the same structure and use exactly the same acupuncture points or cosmic batteries for the correction procedure.

Hand over the navel

When a palm is placed over the navel, the various *test points* relating to each *meridian* are *touch localised*. The hand over the navel allows the practitioner to access information non-verbally on all the meridians by testing only one muscle.

Healing crisis

See *healing process*.

Healing process

As a result of *energy work*, changes occur that may enable the body to release toxic substances, repair and rebuild tissues and utilize previously inaccessible nutrients. This can lead the client to experience temporary symptoms such as tiredness, headaches, digestive problems, increased sweating and aches and pains. Existing symptoms can appear to become worse. These reactions are not harmful, but are part of the body's healing mechanism.

HK menu

HK does not have specific techniques for specific symptoms, but has a list of techniques and procedures which are broken down into five sub-categories: *energy correction factors, energy toning factors, energy redirection factors, environmental factors* and *adjunctive factors*.

HK tested issue

An issue to be addressed that is identified solely through muscle testing. This may or may not be the same problem or goal that the client is most concerned about. Compare *client specified issue*.

Holding acupuncture points

Reflex points on the *meridians* are held to regulate energy flow. They are held during the *initial balance* and also for *corrections*. Although referred to as points, usually held by touching with fingertips, some of the reflexes are over larger areas that are covered by a hand. See *reflex points*. Compare *cosmic batteries*.

Holding points

See *holding acupuncture points*.

Homeopathic remedy

Homeopathic remedies are traditionally prepared by vigorously shaking a sample of a substance in water. The water is then diluted and vigorously shaken again. This is repeated until only the 'memory' or recording of its energy pattern remains in the water. The exact number of times this process is repeated gives the different homeopathic potencies. The remedies can also be prepared using a homeopathic potentizing machine. The homeopathic remedy for a particular symptom is the one that would cause the symptom if a physical dose of the remedy were given. In HK homeopathic remedies are used in *energy corrections* and are also taken in the traditional way. *Test kits* usually contain homeopathic versions of the test substances.

Homeostatic mechanism

The dynamic process whereby the internal environment of the physical body is maintained within strict limits in order to ensure correct cellular functioning.

Homework

What the client does between sessions, which can include taking nutritional supplements or *flower remedies*, wearing a specific *crystal*, and following an exercise, *rest* or diet plan. Homework is either an *adjunctive factor* or an *energy toning factor*.

I Item correction

See *NV(I) item*.

Imperative correction

A type of *energy correction* that is part of the sub-category *psychological corrections*. Each item is a command or a plea.

Indicator muscle

Any convenient muscle that is tested while *asking verbal questions* or *touch localising*.

Individuality

A fundamental principal of HK is that each person is an individual. The HK practitioner does not use set procedures for particular problems, symptoms or illnesses, but finds the most appropriate work through verbal questioning and muscle testing.

Initial balance

This is an essential preliminary to every HK session. The acupuncture energy system is balanced so that accurate answers to verbal questions can be obtained.

Issue

See *issue title*.

Issue analysis

See *issue title* and *facet analysis*. Compare also *meridian analysis*, *meta analysis* and *overall body sequence*.

Issue title

A precisely worded title for the body of work concerning a particular goal or problem. It is determined by muscle testing. See *client specified issue* and *HK tested issue*.

Item

One single *correction* or *energy toning* activity or *adjunctive* or *energy redirection*. Correction items are very often grouped together. See *group*.

Item sequence

See *overall body sequence*.

Life Transformer

A proprietary device developed by Dr Jimmy Scott. Life transformers are based on gemstones that have been energy-modified to carry permanently a particular psychological or energy- protective quality. There are specific life transformers for specific problems. Life Transformers can be worn or used in *energy corrections* in order to rebalance some particular aspect of the client.

Linked opposite correction

A type of *energy correction* that is part of the sub-category *psychological corrections*. Each item is a phrase consisting of two words linked by 'and'. The first word is positive in nature and the other opposes it in some way, e.g. worthy and degraded.

Locked muscle

When a muscle tests strong. If a verbal question has been asked, this response usually means 'yes'. If the muscle is incapable of unlocking, this may indicate physical damage to the muscle, or *over energy* in the associated meridian.

Magnet test

If the acupuncture system is balanced, the north-seeking pole of a magnet will weaken or unlock the muscle when placed over the belly of the muscle. Using *hand over the navel*, the magnet can be placed over the belly of any muscle, and the indicator will weaken if the meridian system is in balance. The south-seeking pole will strengthen it again. See *confirmation tests*.

Mechanism control

A type of *energy correction* in the *energy control system* subcategory. There are four sub-categories: feeling, experiencing, knowing and behaving. Mechanism control corrections are believed to unblock cell receptor sites.

Menu of techniques and procedures

See *HK menu*

Meridian

The traditional pathways of the body containing *Ch'i* energy. There are twelve bilateral meridians plus two meridians that run up the midline of the body. Most of the meridians are named after an associated organ with which they connect, e.g. kidney meridian. In kinesiology the energy in the meridians is influenced by *holding acupuncture points* on the surface of the body.

Meridian analysis

A way of organizing the work to be done on a client, looking at which specific meridians are not functioning properly either on their own or in relation to other meridians. Compare also *issue analysis, meta analysis* and *overall body sequence*.

Meta analysis

A way of organizing the work to be done on a client, using the concepts of *subtle bodies* as a framework. Compare also *issue analysis, meridian analysis* and *overall body sequence*.

NV (I) Item correction

A type of *energy correction* that is part of the sub-category *psychological corrections*. Each item is a phrase beginning with 'I', e.g. 'I can't be slim.'

Overall body sequence

When the energy system chooses to work in menu sequence rather than according to a named issue. Compare *issue analysis, meta analysis* and *meridian analysis*. Also known as *item sequence*.

Over energy

When the meridian system is disturbed, energy flow is disrupted, so an *element* may be 'starved' of energy, or in other words be in a state of *under energy*. Another part of the system will then be in over energy. During the *initial balance* and when *corrections* are carried out this imbalance is rectified.

Permission

See *conscious permission* and *energy permission*.

Phantom sensation correction

Phantom sensations occur when a part of the body is removed, but the person experiences it as though it is still present. A type of *energy correction* in the *energy control system* sub-category. Also known as phantom limb sensation, although a limb is not always involved.

Phobia

An extremely strong, irrational fear. HK has a specific psychological procedure for phobias.

Pinch test

When a muscle is pinched along its fibres, it will weaken; when stretched or smoothed out, it will strengthen again. The pinch test is used to establish that the indicator muscle is functioning correctly. It is also used as part of the confirmation *tests*.

Pinch/unpinch

See *pinch test*.

Predictions

HK practitioners do not make predictions; they make *projections*.

Priority

Priority does not equal importance. The matter that takes priority is simply the first thing that is required.

Priority issue

The first issue to be addressed, established solely by muscle testing. This may or may not be the same as the client's primary concern. Even when it is the same, the wording of the issue may not obviously relate to the client's symptoms or goals. See *HK Tested Issue*.

Projections

Sometimes the HK practitioner will project what will happen to the client as a result of the treatment. This is a projection (based on everything going forward as expected) and not a prediction (based on being able to see into the future).

Psychological correction

A type of *energy correction* in which the person has to think something stressful while *acupuncture points* are held or *cosmic batteries* are placed on the body. This removes the stress triggered by that particular thought.

Reflex points

When the correct combination of acupuncture points is activated by touch, a balancing reflex is triggered in the energy system. A physiological response, may also be triggered, e.g. neurolymphatic reflex points increase lymph flow. See *holding acupuncture points*.

Relaxation

One of the *adjunctive* factors. Doing something that gives a respite from work and worry. It can involve listening to music, watching television, and so on. Compare *rest*.

Rest

One of the *adjunctive* factors. Rest involves sitting or lying in a comfortable position and doing nothing physically or mentally. Compare *relaxation*.

Robust

A term used in relation to *energy corrections*, which implies that when the correction is completed it is extremely resistant to breaking down.

Scar correction

A type of *energy correction* in the *energy control system* sub-category. The client will touch part of a physical body scar while the system is rebalanced.

SEF

See *sensory energy functioning*.

Sensory energy functioning

A type of *energy correction* in the *energy flow balancing* sub-category. Concerned with making sure that physical sensory information is transmitted to the brain as effectively as possible.

SET

See *symbiotic energy transformation*.

Spin

As *energy* flows through the system, it rotates or spins. Disruptions to the normal spin can cause a proliferation of cells, reduced healing ability, and so on. Some proprietary devices and *life transformers* work to counteract spin problems.

Spin correction

A type of *energy correction* in the *energy control system* sub-category. Concerned with rectifying *spin* problems.

Stressor

Anything that tends to disrupt normal balance or function.

Subtle bodies

Traditionally, six subtle bodies are recognized (etheric, emotional, mental, causal, intuitive and spiritual). They are as much part of the individual as the physical body. They are progressively less physical and more spiritual. *Meta analysis* works directly with these subtle bodies.

Subtle energy

Subtle energy is a loose term used to describe any energy that is not recognized and categorized by conventional scientific knowledge.

Subtle energy bodies

See *subtle bodies*.

Surrogate testing

The muscle of one person, who is balanced, is used to test for information about another person, while the two people are physically touching each other. This is particularly useful for testing small children, anyone who is frail and the mentally handicapped. It can also be used to test animals.

Symbiotic energy transformation (SET)

A type of *energy correction* dealing with *energy mismatch*, *allergy* or *tolerance* problems.

Tapping

See *allergy tap* and *tolerance tap*.

TEB

See *tissue energy block*.

Test kit

A collection of *energy patterns*, kept in small vials, which can be used for allergy and other testing and correcting procedures, e.g. foods, hormones, bacteria, body biochemicals. See also *homeopathic remedies*. A wide range of test kits is available to kinesiology students and practitioners from the author.

Thymus tap

A quick way to balance the *acupuncture meridians*. The area around the thymus (in the upper chest) is tapped in a counter clockwise direction for about thirty seconds.

Time window

A precise period of time during which certain energy procedures must be completed. Time windows are established through muscle testing.

Tissue energy block

A type of *energy correction* in which the client is required to place their hands on their own body. It is concerned with energy blockages within tissues, which may have resulted from physical trauma or other disturbances. There is usually a nutrient blockage in the area that it being touched by the client.

TL'ing

See *touch localising*.

Tolerance

With *allergy* any amount of a substance will disturb the client's energy system, but with tolerance the client's energy system is only disturbed when the client exceeds a tolerance level for that substance. This is unique to the individual and will vary in response to stress, and so on.

Tolerance correction

A type of *energy correction* that increases the level of a substance that someone can be exposed to without the energy system becoming unbalanced. There are two ways of doing this: *symbiotic energy transformation* or *tolerance tap*.

Tolerance tap

A *tolerance correction* involving tapping specific points on the body and simultaneously holding specific areas while the substance is placed on the body.

Touch localising

An *indicator muscle* is tested while simultaneously a specific *reflex point* or area on the client is touched. This is an alternative way of gathering information to *asking verbal questions*. HK practitioners also use touch localising to confirm something already established by verbal questioning.

Under energy

When the meridian system is disturbed, energy flow is disrupted, so an *element* may be 'starved' of energy or in a state of under energy. Another part of the system will then be in *over energy*. During the *initial balance* and when *corrections* are carried out this imbalance is rectified.

Unlocked muscle

When the muscle tests weak in response to an energy stress. If a verbal question has been asked, this usually means 'no'. If the muscle is incapable of locking, this may indicate physical damage to the muscle, or *under energy* in the associated meridian.

Verbal questioning

See *asking verbal questions*.

Visualization

An *energy toning* factor involving the person repeatedly and vividly visualizing some desired outcome as though it has already been achieved. The appropriate visualization is established through muscle testing. Some *energy corrections* may also have a visualization component.

Word lists

Compilation of words used in corrections. The practitioner can use muscle testing to find the appropriate word or phrase on a list for an item.

Yang

Yang and *yin* represent opposite aspects of existence, which in coming together form a unified and balanced whole. Yang qualities include expansiveness, dryness, masculinity, lightness, heat and hollowness, but nothing is entirely yang or entirely yin.

Yes/no

When the energy system is in balance, saying or thinking 'no' will weaken the indicator muscle. Saying 'yes' strengthens the muscle or switches it back on. See *confirmation tests*.

Yin

Yin and *yang* represent opposite aspects of existence, which, in coming together, form a unified and balanced whole. Yin qualities include femininity, receptivity, darkness, coolness and solidity, but nothing is entirely yin or entirely yang.

Address Corrections
Finding an HK practitioner in the UK:
www.hk4health.co.uk; 08707 655980

HK training in the UK:
Ann Parker, 01246 862339; annparker@lineone.net

Kinesiology Federation:
PO Box 28908, Dalkieth, Edinburgh, EH22 2YQ; 08700 113545